There's Always a Rainbow

She was 28, pregnant with twins and diagnosed with cancer...

Annette Kramer's story as told to Michelle H. Kramer

First published by AuthorHouse 04/12/04

ISBN: 1-4140-6733-X (e-book)
ISBN: 1-4184-3198-2 (Paperback)

Library of Congress Control Number: 2004091302

Printed in the United States of America
Bloomington, IN

This book is printed on acid free paper.

Dedication:

This book is dedicated to Annette.
It's her story, in her words.
All I did was put it on paper. She lived it.
May we all learn from it.

INTRODUCTION

Once upon a time in West Valley, Utah, there lived a beautiful young girl named Annette. She grew up and met her Prince Charming, David, who happened to be an LDS missionary from Michigan. After his mission, he returned to Utah and proposed. They were married for time and eternity in the Salt Lake Temple and lived happily ever after.....

Not.

Fairy tales are not without their problems.

CHAPTER ONE

"I Have *What?*"

"I'm sorry, Annette. You have cancer."

The doctor's words took my breath away. At age 28, and seven months into a pregnancy with twins, the word 'cancer' was the last thing I expected to hear. Tears welled up in my eyes. I blinked them back while focusing on the dots in the ceiling of the recovery room. Cancer! At that moment everything became a blur. I kept hearing the echo of that word -- *cancer*-- over and over in my mind. How could this happen to me? The numbness of shock washed over me as my husband David appeared by my side to hold my hand. His eyes were swollen and red; his cheeks wet as he looked into my face. Neither of us knew what lay ahead.

But, as usual, I'm getting ahead of myself so let me start back at the beginning. David and I lived in West Jordan, Utah with our two little girls, Angie (age 6) and Jessica (age 2). In June of 1991, I was not feeling well. I was sick to my stomach and tired all of the time. All I wanted to do was sleep. I wondered if I had mononucleosis or something. The thought occurred to me that I might be pregnant. I've always had a real irregular cycle anyway so I couldn't be sure. I went to the doctor's office for a pregnancy test and they said, "Well, we can't really tell if it's negative or positive. Come back in another week and we'll test you again." I quickly determined I didn't have patience to wait that long. "No," I told the nurse, "I think I'll run over to the hospital for a blood test. I can't stand not knowing for sure." I knew that blood tests were more accurate and could detect pregnancy earlier than a urine test.

I went on over to the hospital and gave them some blood. The nurse came out a few minutes later smiling, "Congratulations Annette. You're pregnant!"

I guess the shock showed on my face. I gasped, "Really??"

She frowned, "Aren't you happy?"

"I guess so...." I sighed, "this pregnancy wasn't planned. I'm not too sure how my husband is going to take it."

Let's just say David wasn't exactly thrilled. But I had hopes that over the next few months the idea would grow on him.

I eagerly looked forward to my first appointment with Dr. Baker. I had no idea how far along I was or when my due date would be. My mom worked for Dr. Baker so I chatted with her for a few minutes before the nurse took me back to the exam room. I was feeling queasy so I laid down on the exam table to wait.

Several minutes later Dr. Baker came in and performed all of the usual measurements, and exams. "Well Annette," he said sounding surprised, "by the size of your uterus I'd say you're about 12 weeks along already!"

I was shocked, "You're kidding! You mean I've made it through my first trimester without even knowing I was pregnant? Cool!"

But over the next two months I only gained two pounds and I wasn't getting any higher in uterine centimeters. Dr. Baker remarked, "Well, we thought you were due around December 10th and I am retiring on December 31. I want to send you for an ultrasound to make sure we've calculated correctly. If you're really not due until January, then I'll refer you to another doctor."

I really wanted *him* to deliver my baby. I thought it would be kind of neat if the last baby he ever delivered was mine. I went right over for the ultrasound. I laid on the table waiting for the technician to arrive. I looked at the monitor beside me and thought it was interesting how this machine could show me my baby while it was still inside of me. *Is it too early to tell if it's a boy or a girl?* I wondered. David had mentioned he'd like to know the sex of this one ahead of time if possible.

The tech came in, switched off the light and pulled a stool over to sit on. The faint glow from the screen illuminated the room. I heard the clock ticking on the wall. She squirted some warm gel on my stomach and placed the ultrasound scope on it. She moved it around as she looked intently at the screen. "So you know you're having twins?"

I nearly fell off the table. "I'm *what?*" I exclaimed.

She giggled apologetically, "I'm sorry Annette! I assumed you already knew!" She pointed at the screen. "Look, you're having twins. And I think....they're both boys."

I was struck dumb. *Oh my gosh. I don't believe this! Twins!*

When she finished the scan she handed me some tissues to wipe the gel off my stomach. "Could you possibly print out a picture for me?" I asked. "My husband is *never* going to believe this without proof!"

She chuckled again. "Sure Annette. You go on out in the waiting room. I'll bring you one in a few minutes."

I found a seat beside an older woman. I'm sure she thought I was retarded because I couldn't wipe the stupid grin off my face. She smiled at me and asked if I was getting an ultrasound because I was pregnant. I found myself blurting out, "I'm having TWINS! And you're the first person I've told and I don't even know you!"

She started laughing. "Well honey, you're going to have your hands full!"

That proved to be the understatement of the century.

I drove home with my heart jumping a mile a minute. I could not believe I was pregnant *with twins*. It was so unreal. I couldn't wait to tell David. But I wanted to tell him in person because I just *had* to see the expression on his face. Of course I couldn't keep news like this to myself so by the time David got home I'd already told *everybody else* in the family!!

I heard the door open and close when he came home that afternoon. He walked up the stairs, into the kitchen. I was trying to act very casual.

"Um... I had my ultrasound today." I said working very hard to contain the excitement in my voice.

He picked up a pile of mail sitting on the counter and began sorting through it. "Umm hmmm...." he glanced up at me with a blank expression like "So?"

"Do you want to know what we're having?" I teased. I was enjoying dragging it out like this because I knew he had NO CLUE what was coming.

"Yeah, sure," he answered distractedly. I tried to get his full attention.

"I think you better sit down," I told him.

He paused briefly to look up from the mail and grinned, "Why? Cause it's another girl?"

"Noooo.... really, I think you better sit down. I mean it." I convinced him I wasn't going to tell him until he sat down so he pulled the chair out from the table, slumped down in it and looked at me expectantly.

"Okay. I'm sitting. Now tell me."

"We're having *twin boys*."

He burst out laughing! He didn't believe me! He was sure I was kidding because I'm such a joker. So I said it a little more firmly, "David, *really*, we're having twin boys." He still would NOT believe me!

I reached into my purse and pulled out the ultrasound picture to show him both babies. *That* finally convinced him. Then he became pretty excited. He acted like he was Mr. Stud -- you know -- fathering two sons at the same time. But later, when he was reading a book about twins he learned that it had nothing to do with *him*. He got kind of ruffled, "Well, wait a sec. You mean it's not because I'm Superman or anything?"

"Ooops, sorry to disappoint you, honey." I chuckled.

We were talking one night about complications that can arise with twins like premature labor. I was on my feet a lot because I am a beautician and I do people's hair at home. I usually made the car payment with the money I earned. "You know Annette," David said with concern, "if you end up having to go down in bed, then you won't be doing hair for awhile. Maybe we should sell the car."

"We can do that," I said, "but you can't leave me stranded at home. Buy me something. I don't care what it costs or what shape it's in. As long as it gets me from point A to point B. I just can't stand not having any car at all."

He began scanning the newspaper ads and a few weeks later he bought me a used station wagon. He got a good deal on it. And even though it was butt ugly... I was very happy to have it!

I planned on having to go on bed rest when I reached about seven months. I booked a lot of perms and haircuts to try to save up some money and as luck would have it, I made myself go into labor.

One night after I'd had a very busy day of doing hair I climbed into bed beside David. My feet were swollen and my back hurt. Suddenly I felt a tingling sensation in my stomach. *Must be Braxton Hicks contractions*, I told myself. Then I remembered my sister-in-law had real labor pains that felt like tingling. I waited a few minutes and it happened a second time. Five minutes later, the same thing. *Oh great!*

"David -- I think I'm in labor."

"No, you're not," he mumbled sleepily.

"I'm having these really weird tingling things every five minutes."

"I thought labor pains hurt," he grumbled.

"Hon, trust me. We'd better go to the hospital."

I was only 29 weeks along. My new OB, Dr. Mark Curtis, (since I was now considered a high risk pregnancy, Dr. Baker couldn't deliver me) was able to stop the contractions with medication. He sent me home and put me on complete bed rest. I cancelled the rest of my booked hair appointments. Taking care of the babies was now my top priority. I never realized how fragile life was until I saw how my innocent actions affected what happened to those babies who were completely dependent upon me for their very lives. It was a scary realization.

At 5 foot 1 inches and 100 pounds I wasn't sure if I could even carry two babies at once.

Where could they go? There wasn't that much room! I soon learned that these boys would make room. They managed to get all the space they needed while I struggled for air and suffered bruised ribs from their kicking! It was so uncomfortable, but I didn't complain because it was so thrilling to think about how things would be after they were born. I knew I'd have my hands full -- thankfully I was still in the dark concerning everything I'd have to handle in the near future.

I asked David's brother Steve to give me a blessing that everything would be okay with my babies. As he began the blessing he started telling me that I was going to need a lot of help in the coming months. He talked about how I was willing to give to others but would have to humble myself in order to accept all the help I would need. He went on and on about the assistance I'd be getting and I remember thinking, *These twins must be really bad! They must be twins from hell because I'm gonna need all this help!* When he was through, Steve commented that he felt that was one of the strangest blessings he'd ever given. Little did he know he had truly revealed a prophetic warning of things to come.

I had been performing breast exams regularly because earlier in the year my obstetrician had said, "Annette, there's a little teeny thing like a piece of sand in your breast. It's not very big but I want you to check it and make sure it's not getting bigger." He showed me where it was, and he didn't seem overly concerned about it. I was conscientious to follow his instructions so I checked it often. Usually I couldn't even feel anything there. I figured it was nothing.

I was 33 weeks along in my pregnancy and my boobs were growing along with everything else. As I was doing my self exam I felt what seemed like pea-sized lumps. *Hmmm, that's strange,* I thought. *These aren't in the same place as Dr. Curtis said. These are more to the side and up toward my armpit.* I kept checking them, wondering if I was imagining it. But they were easy to find. There was no mistaking that something was there, but what was it?

The next day was Thanksgiving. I knew my doctor wouldn't be able to see me until after the holiday so I tried not to think about it. But you know what happens when you try *not* to think about something? That's all you think about! I tried telling myself it was a plugged milk duct or something pregnancy related. I hoped that was all it was, but there was a nagging suspicion in the back of my mind. *Could it be cancer?* I was only 28 years old! *Cancer doesn't happen to women that young, does it? I'm pregnant with twins -- Heavenly Father wouldn't take me away from them, would He? Cancer doesn't run in my family, so how could I possibly have it?* These thoughts ran through my mind in never ending circles.

A few days later I was in the obstetricians' office pointing out the lumps I had found. He didn't comment on them directly but when he finished the exam he asked me to make sure I stopped by the front desk.

"Hi, I'm here to make my next appointment," I told the receptionist.

"Are you Annette Kramer?" she asked.

"Yes," I replied.

"Dr. Curtis asked me to let you know he scheduled an appointment for you to see a surgeon on Wednesday. He wants to run a biopsy on those cysts. Here is his name and address and the time of the appointment." She handed me a card.

A surgeon! Again, the thought crossed my mind that it could be cancer, but I still told myself, *Aw, God wouldn't let that happen to me.*

That night when I talked to my sister I found out that my maternal grandmother had had a mastectomy. I *did* have a family history of breast cancer.

I felt my heart pounding with fear.

I met with Dr. Jack, a surgeon at Cottonwood Hospital in Murray, a few days later for the biopsy.

"I'm only 28." I pointed out. "Aren't I too young to have cancer?"

"I just had a really young patient with breast cancer," he told me. "She was 33 years old and she was also pregnant. She had to have a double mastectomy. Does cancer run in your family?"

That's when I told him about my grandmother. She died when I was 20 years old and prior to that she had served a lot of church missions so I hadn't spent much time with her. Whether or not she had a breast was never a topic of conversation I'd had with her as a child. I did know that she used to stuff a sock in her bra… but I just used to think, *Ha! Grandma's stuffin' her bra!* I didn't wonder why.

My biopsy was done as an outpatient procedure using a local anesthetic. For some reason I didn't numb up like I should have so I felt quite a bit of it. They couldn't put me under general anesthesia because I was pregnant and it was too risky for the babies. He took a couple little pieces, sent it directly to the lab and had them rush the results. By the time I was wheeled into recovery he had arrived to give me the bad news. "I'm sorry Annette, you have cancer."

My heart quickened. My hands protectively clutched my stomach. In one way I was so full of life. How could my body now rebel against me? *The lumps are cancerous. I could die. Oh my gosh, what do I do now?* This was unbelievable. David and I cried a long time. I had never known anyone dealing with breast cancer. I had no idea what I was facing. Trying to lighten the mood I joked to David, "Oh well. I'll just have to get a better 'set.'" We laughed but the situation was still very hard to deal with.

David asked me, "Annette . . . how do you feel about all this?" I knew he meant spiritually.

I thought for few minutes and replied, "I'm sure I'll be okay. I know Heavenly Father

19

wouldn't do this to me. He wouldn't let me die."

I know that God doesn't *do* this to people, but I was hoping the odds were for me, you know -- 28 years old, pregnant with twins.... I mean how many cases have you ever heard of a women having breast cancer that young and pregnant with twins? I learned that at that time I set the record at Cottonwood Hospital for being the youngest person diagnosed with breast cancer. Gee... give me a medal.

My surgeon walked directly over to my OB's office after the procedure, still in his surgical scrubs and everything. They talked for a long time trying to decide what to do. Knowing he went over so fast made me realize this might be worse than I thought.

When I got home I called one of my sisters to tell her. I got out the words, "I have cancer," and then I started crying so hard I couldn't talk and had to hang up. My little girl, Jessica was on the bed beside me and she began bawling because I was. We were both crying so hard we became hysterical and David finally took her out of the room. She was just a few months away from turning 3 years old but she could sense something bad was happening. So in the future, when I was having a really tough time and I needed to cry, I would go to the back of my walk-in closet, sit on the hamper, and let it out. Then, when I was better, I'd come out. It was just too hard on the girls to see me cry. I couldn't permit that.

CHAPTER TWO

"Drop dead! Eat dirt!"

In keeping with the old adage, "When it rains, it pours," the next week was horrible. A friend of mine who suffered from Chronic Fatigue syndrome contracted pneumonia and died. David got into an accident with the company truck -- thankfully he wasn't seriously hurt. He had a mild case of whiplash. My father-in-law was undergoing eye surgery. Both he and his wife were worried they might lose their jobs in January due to layoffs. The last straw

"Drop dead! Eat dirt!"

happened one night as we laid in our waterbed --- it collapsed to the floor at about 1:00 in the morning. We just laughed and laughed.

Suddenly it seemed that everywhere I turned, the topic of cancer was staring me in the face. October had been National Breast Cancer Awareness month. The TV had been broadcasting reports, commercials and commentaries all month concerning breast cancer. That is probably what caused me to find the lumps when I did -- those things reminded me to do the exam.

The cancer board at the hospital reviewed my case and decided it was best to wait until the twins were born before doing anything. They wanted me to try to keep the babies in for three more weeks. At that time I would be 36 weeks which they felt was far enough along for the babies to have a good chance at being healthy. I spent the next three weeks in my bed, scared to death of what lay ahead. I often prayed, *Heavenly Father, what if I die? Who would raise my children? I want to mother my babies. I want to be here for my kids.* I didn't think David couldn't handle a 6-year old, 2-year old and newborn twins by himself.....*How could this happen to me? Why would You let this happen? What's the purpose?*

I found an answer to that last question in a song by Janice Kapp Perry. These words became my philosophy, helping me put my cancer experience in perspective. They played

"Drop dead! Eat dirt!"
through my mind many times over the following
months and years:

Tell me friend, why are you blind?
Why doesn't He who worked the miracles send light into your eyes?
Tell me friend, if you understand
Why doesn't He with power to raise the dead, just make you whole again?
It would be so easy for Him. I watch you and in sorrow question Why?
Then you my friend, in perfect faith reply:

Chorus:
Didn't He say he sent us to be tested?
Didn't He say the way would not be sure?
But didn't He say we could live with Him
Forevermore, well and whole. If we but patiently endure?
After the trial, we will be blessed. But this life is the test.

Tell me friend, I see your pain
Why when you pray in faith for healing, does the crippling thorn remain?
Help me see if you understand
Why doesn't He who healed the lame man come
With healing in His wings?
It would be so easy for Him. I watch you and in sorry question Why?
Then you my friend in perfect faith reply:

Chorus
Didn't He say he sent us to be tested?
Didn't He say the way would not be sure?
But didn't He say we could live with Him
Forevermore, well and whole. If we but patiently endure?
After the trial, we will be blessed. But this life is the test.

There's Always a Rainbow

Tell me love, why must you die?
Why must your loved ones stand with empty arms
And ask the question, WHY?
Help me know, so I can go on
Why, when your love and faith sustained me can this precious
gift be gone?
From the depths of sorrow I cry!
Though pains of grief within my soul arise....
The whispering of the Spirit stills my cries.....

Chorus
Didn't He say he sent us to be tested?
Didn't He say the way would not be sure?
But didn't He say we could live with Him
Forevermore, well and whole. If we but patiently endure?
After the trial, we will be blessed. But this life is the test.

Copywrite (c) 1985Janice Kapp Perry
Used by Permission

After being told I had cancer it came as no
surprise that I was hungry for knowledge. I went
to the library and to several bookstores looking
for books about breast cancer. What I found
was extremely disappointing. First of all, the
majority of books were depressing. The authors
were mostly concerned with how deformed
and maimed they had become. Others were

angry and their bitterness shot off the page at me, which was distressing. All of the authors were much older than I was. They didn't have small children at home or even children at all. I noticed a lot of the women didn't believe in God, or had different religious backgrounds than I did. I wanted to read a book written by a member of my own church, someone who had the same belief system and gospel knowledge that I had. I needed a book that made me feel *better*, not hopeless! But at that time, I didn't find anything.

One afternoon I was reading my patriarchal blessing and a sentence in it seemed to literally jump off the page at me. It said, "You have much to tell the world" and then it counseled me to be sure to write things down and keep a journal. That's when I had a really strong impression that I needed to write my story down. I don't know exactly what I have to tell the world, but I hope that I can offer words of hope, encouragement and peace to someone else who might be going through this same ordeal. I think attitude is very important.

I started looking at my life differently. I tried to see the "big picture" that God sees. We live here on earth with such a narrow perspective. We're so busy caught up in paying bills, working, cooking, cleaning, daily chores, entertainment, and so on that we don't see what life is *really* all about. The plan of salvation takes on such a deeper meaning when you know you could die sooner than you expected.

It was now the end of December and I was so tired of bed rest. I *rolled* myself out of the bed (don't laugh, I was as big as a house) a few days after Christmas to go a family gathering.

"What do you think you're doing Annette?" David asked.

"Drop dead! Eat dirt!"

"I'm going to moms' for the party." I told him.

"Don't you think that's a bad idea? What if you go into labor?"

I looked down to find where my feet were so I could slide my shoes on but I couldn't see them over my enormous stomach. I sat on the edge of the bed feeling like a beached whale. "Dr. Curtis said I was dilated about 4 centimeters when I saw him last. I'll be 36 weeks along tomorrow so if anything happens I think it's okay."

"If you say so," David replied reluctantly.

I WANTED labor to start -- I was SO uncomfortable. My cousin's husband had seen me the day before and said to her, "I have never seen anybody so big in my whole life! Annette is HUGE." And he was right!

Well, I had fun at the party but it was short-lived. After a little while I began to feel terrible.

We stayed until 9:00 pm, then I turned to David and said, "I'm sorry but I can't do this anymore. I have to go home." We went to pick up the kids. I couldn't even breathe because I had babies squishing my insides. I also had a very painful ear infection and was on an antibiotic. I was pretty miserable. A little after midnight I had my first pain and thought, *Oh no! I cannot do labor with an ear infection, it hurts too much. I don't want to do this tonight. Just let me sleep!*

But five minutes later I had another one. I called my brother because we'd arranged for him to stay with the girls when I went into labor, especially if it was at night. Five minutes later I called my mom and said, "Make sure he gets here and doesn't get into an accident or anything because we cannot wait one more minute to go to the hospital." She said okay, so we left the door unlocked for him and took off for the hospital. The girls were sound asleep and he lived only a few minutes away so we felt confident everything would be okay and it was.

We got to the hospital a little after 1:00 am. They put me in the pre-labor room and the nurse checked me. "Whoa! You're dilated 7 centimeters! I think you'll be going into the delivery room *right now.*"

I didn't want a delivery room. "Can't I have a birthing suite? I'm having these babies naturally." I said.

"I'm afraid not," the nurse replied, "twins are born in a delivery room, just in case we run into complications."

Bummer.

When I reached the delivery room a few minutes later I commented, "Oh, so *this* is what a delivery room looks like!"

The nurse asked, "How many children have you had?"

"Well, this is my third pregnancy," I explained, "but I've always gone so fast I never made it into a delivery room or a birthing suite. I always end up delivering in the labor room." I noticed she moved quite a bit faster after I told her that.

My labor progressed rapidly and surprisingly it wasn't very painful. I guess with twins my uterus couldn't contract as hard because it was so stretched out. I was breathing through the contractions and David was dying of shock. He'd ask me, "Are you having a contraction now?" I'd answer very calmly that "Yes," I was. I think he expected me to be screaming twice as loud. He'd seen me in labor twice before and I was *not* kind!

"Okay, Annette, we're ready. Push!" instructed Dr. Curtis.

"Come on! You can do it -- push!" encouraged the nurse.

"Drop dead! Eat dirt!"

I bore down and suddenly little Scott entered the world. It was 1:59am. They quickly put him on the scale and called out *4 pounds 9 ounces!*

"Okay Annette, go ahead and push again," the doctor ordered.

Have you ever thought about how that would be? I mean... you just had a baby and you think *oh good... it's over.* And then the doctor tells you that you have to do it AGAIN??

Push again? I thought. *Drop dead! Eat dirt! No way!* Out loud I whined, "Can't I just do this tomorrow?"

He laughed at me and said, "Uh, that's probably not a good idea. I tell you what -- if you push this baby out I'll send your husband down the hall to get you a milkshake." That sounded pretty good to me, so at 2:11 a.m. Shane arrived. He was a healthy 4 lbs. 12 oz.

They took me into a maternity recovery room. I'd never been in one of those either. We didn't have maternity insurance, and when they put me into the recovery room I just laid there worrying that I was being charged for it and I just wanted to go to my regular room!

People kept coming in and asking me "Are you the one who delivered twins naturally with no anesthetic??" I didn't understand what the big deal was. I had *all* my kids naturally and the twins hurt the least! I didn't realize I was such a novelty. I think I hurt more AFTER the birth than during. The doctor was stitching me up and I was still having contractions because of the Pitocin they were giving me so I begged for a pain shot. They gave me one, but they must have hit a nerve because I felt it for 3 months afterward! Every time I walked down the stairs I could feel pain.

Right after I delivered, the nurse asked me if I wanted to breast feed my babies and I told her, "I can't. I have breast cancer." *That* news traveled around the hospital in record time! Nurses from all over were stopping by to see me. They couldn't believe this young mother could have just given birth to twins *and* be dealing with breast cancer at the same time. I was having trouble believing it myself, and I was living it!

As I said before, we didn't have insurance so I went home 12 hours after delivery. It was weird to leave without the babies. The hospital went ahead and admitted them to keep them overnight just to be safe. I was actually relieved to get a good night's sleep. I felt like I had been hit by a truck. I was completely wiped out.

CHAPTER THREE

"Pain and panic attacks"

Once I got home I crashed. I'd had weeks of emotional stress, given birth, and was on painkillers. When Dr. Jack, my surgeon, called me at my house I thought I was dreaming. I don't remember much about the conversation except his voice saying "Annette! Are you there Annette?" I couldn't comprehend anything; I was so groggy. Finally I confessed, "I'm sorry. I don't understand what you're saying."

"Okay. Repeat after me," he said, "I'll come see you..."

"I'll come see you...."

"Monday at three."

"Monday at three..."

That was all I could remember and I wasn't sure if I hallucinated it or not. I went ahead into his office on Monday and he completely floored me by announcing, "You're going into surgery tomorrow at one o'clock."

"Tomorrow?" I gasped, "I just gave birth two days ago!"

He answered gravely, "I know that, but we can't wait any longer."

So just three days after giving birth to the twins I went back to the hospital for surgery. I didn't even know what would be happening. I just assumed my breast was going to be cut off. I didn't ask a lot of questions at that time. I wasn't really sure *what* to ask.

Everything happened so quickly that I didn't have time to prepare and I didn't know what to expect. My life felt out of control. David came to the hospital with me. I kissed him goodbye and they wheeled me back towards the operating room but then they parked me in the hall! There was *nobody* there with me. I was completely terrified. Here I was, a young person with breast cancer, and anyone with breast cancer is going to be terrified whether they're young or not, but I was all by myself and frightened. I just wanted to cry. People walked by me and it was like I wasn't even there. No one looked at me. It was the weirdest feeling. I was so alone. And that was the most horrible thing -- to feel that way. I was totally alone and wasn't prepared for it. I didn't feel the Spirit or anything. It was like even God had left me. Finally the anesthesiologist came and put me out -- right there in the hall! I didn't see my doctor, or the operating room, or anything. It was the coldest, most awful experience. I felt like a piece of meat. I'm sure it was because I didn't have time to prepare myself. I wasn't given time to catch my breath between giving birth, running tests, and having surgery. It was just boom, boom, boom!

I woke up after the operation with pain surging through my arm and back.

That's strange, I thought, *shouldn't it be my chest hurting?*

"David," I said, "I think they cut me all the way through my back!"

"Annette, they didn't cut you all the way through your back, "he assured me. "They removed the mammary gland, the lumps, and a bunch of lymph nodes."

"Yes they did!" I insisted, "I can feel it!" The pain in my arm and back was so intense I had no strength to move. The nurse came in to give me a pain shot and a foam pad to lay on. They rolled me over and gave me a back massage but the pain *never* went away.

Later that night I woke up to a lot of strange noises. Looking at the clock I saw it was midnight. I could hear fireworks going off and people shouting "Happy New Year!" *Tonight is New Year's Eve*, I realized. I laid there in that hospital room wondering what 1992 would bring for me. I was so afraid. *Please Heavenly Father,* I prayed, *let me live to raise my children.*

The next afternoon I was napping when I experienced something really strange. All of a sudden, I awoke very abruptly. I was filled with intense fear. The hospital room felt dark and icy cold even though I could see through the window shades that it was light outside. My heart pounded rapidly in my chest. I felt the trickle of perspiration down my back. *What is going on? Why am I so afraid?* I looked around the room.

No one was there but I felt the presence of --- something..... What?

The devil?

I knew something was there. An evil presence filled my room. I could *feel* it. *Oh my gosh,* I thought, *I have to get out of here. I have to tell someone. Please Heavenly Father, make it go away!* I felt panic and nausea sweep over me in a wave that left me shaking. I tried to find the buzzer to ring the nurse -- though I had no idea what I'd tell her when she came in. But I couldn't move.

And then, just as suddenly as it had arrived; it was gone.

Peace flooded my mind. My thoughts became calm. My breathing slowed to normal and the muscles in my rigid body relaxed. *Okay --- I'm okay.* I told myself. *It's gone. I probably just imagined it anyway. Oh my gosh, that was weird. I really think the devil was in my room. I guess the stress is taking it's toll...*

I don't understand what that experience meant. But all I can say is that it made a *big* impact on me. I was so scared! But then when it was gone, the peace I felt was so nice and warm and protective. Maybe it was to show me that I had to go through some bad stuff but afterwards things would be really good again. That's what I hoped for anyway.

Even though I had just had breast surgery I was recuperating on the maternity floor because I still needed my post-partum needs attended to. The nurse kept coming in to take my blood pressure out of the arm that they had just stripped the lymph nodes out of! Every time she walked in the room, I'd start bawling. "*Please*, I don't want you to take my blood pressure in that arm!"

She'd just pat me on the arm and say, "Oh honey, we have to. We can't do it in the other arm because there's an IV in it."

This happened several times. Every time a crippling pain rose up from my arm --- each nerve ending sending silent screams throughout my body. I nearly passed out as dizziness overwhelmed me. My stomach would knot up when I saw the blood pressure cuff. Finally the shift of nurses changed.

When the next nurse came in I started sobbing hysterically.

"Don't take my blood pressure!" I begged. I meant it. I was going to refuse to cooperate. They'd have to restrain me to get it.

The nurse looked at me curiously and inquired, "Have they been doing it in your LEFT arm?"

I wailed "YES!"

She looked sick and stunned. "Oh Annette," she consoled, "You are NEVER, *ever*, even after you leave the hospital, forever, the rest of your life --- *never* supposed to have blood pressure taken on that side."

"Then why didn't the other nurses know that?" I cried.

She explained how the other nurses were maternity nurses, so they wouldn't know. She had been a surgery nurse so she knew all about it. She said, "If anybody else comes in and tries to take it in your left arm you tell them to call me or to call the surgery ward because they are *never* supposed to take blood pressure on that side." She posted a big sign above my bed. I didn't have a problem after that.

CHAPTER FOUR

"The Journey Begins"

A few days later my oncologist, Dr. Patricia Legant called me into her office. I had my aunt bring me because I was still on painkillers and couldn't drive. I didn't bother to ask David to come because I didn't know that I was going in for test results. Dr. Legant walked in and dropped a bombshell in my lap. "Annette, you have eight out of fifteen lymph nodes that are cancerous and if you want the chance to live to see your children grow up then I recommend you have a full mastectomy, chemotherapy and radiation." Just at that moment she received a phone call that said she was needed elsewhere immediately. She patted my arm and said, "I'm so sorry I have to drop a bomb on you like that and leave but I'll be right back."

As soon as she'd closed the door I started bawling. I wasn't prepared to hear this. Again the denial crept into my mind, *Oh everything is going to be fine. Yes I have cancer but God wouldn't let...* You know how I kept doing that --- but I stopped doing it after awhile. I thought it wasn't wise. Nobody should presume to know the mind and will of God.

When Dr. Legant came back she told me to go right over and see my surgeon; he was waiting for me. With every step towards his office I became more panicked. I didn't have a clue what I was facing. Realizing this was more serious than I thought, and that I might die was scaring the crap out of me.

Dr. Jack began by explaining all of my "options." "Well, Annette we could take more of your breast and we could do this and we could do that." And I just interrupted him and said, "You know... I don't want to mess around with this. Just take it all off." So an appointment was made for two weeks later to have a mastectomy.

In addition to all of this, we had put our home up for sale soon after we found out we were having twins. Two days before I had the mastectomy we received an offer on the house. So we worked it out that we had two weeks to relocate. I thought it was nice in a way that I wouldn't have to help with the move. Packing and carrying boxes was out because I'd be recovering from surgery. I really hated giving up that house because it was our first home, and we had lots of memories there. But this was definitely a time of change for us. Everything in our lives was upside down -- why should where we live be any different?

I became rather depressed about this time. Who could blame me? I was suffering from the baby blues because I had all these hormones fluctuating in me. I had been through one surgery and was preparing for another. I was scared to do chemotherapy. And I was *really* upset about my hair falling out. It was equally hard to think about losing my breast. And now we had to move out of the one place that offered me some emotional security! I felt like I had to hold it all inside. Well, let me tell you, it's hard to be strong all of the time.

I then learned that before I could have the mastectomy I had to have a bone scan. The doctor said she wanted to make sure the cancer hadn't already spread to my bones. I was freaking out. I knew that if I had bone cancer I might as well kiss my butt goodbye. I remember calling my neighbor Jolene and we were both bawling on the phone. I kept saying, "I know I'm gonna die of bone cancer!" I was really stressed about this because it seemed that *everything* was worse than they thought as they did the tests. I kept thinking *This is it. I'm dead*. The bone scan came back clear. I was so relieved about that. Still… it didn't lessen my other anxieties.

I remembered how awful it felt to be alone when I had my first surgery. I didn't want that to happen again. Every night for two weeks I prayed, *Heavenly Father, please don't let me be alone. Please don't let me cry in front of everybody. I can't handle crying.*

CHAPTER FIVE

"My cups runneth over"

The morning that I was scheduled for surgery, I woke up to discover my breasts were absolutely huge. I got into the shower and once the warm water hit I realized why. I had milk! *But this is impossible,* I thought. *My twins are 2 1/2 weeks old, and they gave me pills to dry me up.* I looked down again. No doubt about it. Boy, oh boy did I have milk. Gallons of it. *Can they do a mastectomy when you have milk?* I wondered.

I got dressed and called the hospital. They said my doctor was in surgery but he would want to talk to me so I better come in. I rode to the hospital making a mental list of all the questions I wanted to ask. This time I was determined not to go into this blindly. I wanted to know exactly what was happening. Were they planning to cut off both of my breasts or just one? What exactly does a "full" mastectomy mean? If you don't know much about breast cancer, these terms are very confusing.

Dr. Jack came in and I told him, "Uh, I think we have a problem. My milk came in."

He chuckled, "That's okay. We'll pack one side in ice and the anesthetic will also help dry you up. It'll be a little messier, but it doesn't matter."

"So I guess there's no getting out of it then?" I asked hopefully.

He looked at me soberly and shook his head no.

"Dr. Jack, are you going to cut off *both* of my breasts?" I asked hesitantly.

"No. We're just taking the one with cancer. The other one is perfectly fine. Are you planning on eventually having reconstruction? Because if you are, I need to know so I can make provisions for that."

"Yes," I answered. "I do want reconstruction."

He nodded. "That's good. You're young and I'm sure you'll be glad you did it."

To my surprise and delight they let David come into the surgical suite with me! I was so shocked because they don't let ANYBODY into that area. But they parked us in this closet thing that had a desk and linens and things for the operating room. It was big, but it was still a closet. Still, I wasn't alone and that was such a relief. My surgeon came in and talked to us for a few minutes. I had seen the chart that said I was having a "Left Modified Radical" and I thought, *Oh my gosh, a RADICAL.* Don't you think the term "modified radical" is like a contradiction????

Then the anesthesiologist came in to put me out. *I was never alone for one second.* The anesthesiologist pushed me to the front of the operating room and everybody was waiting there for me. And right when I went to cry... I just went unconscious. I didn't even get one tear out before I went under. I never had to cry or be alone. It was like Heavenly Father did that for me so I wouldn't have to go through all that fear like I did before. And I thought, *Well, if I have to go through this, at least He's here helping me along the way.*

When I came out of surgery my dad was there. I sometimes felt bad when people were there because I was so groggy. I felt like I should entertain everybody and I couldn't. I had a lot of worries, about the babies and Angie and Jessica. So I said to David, "Go home and be with the babies." Finally he agreed. That night he took care of them by himself and I think he almost had a nervous breakdown! It's not easy!

Actually the twins were not bad -- it's just that caring for them was constant. They got up every two hours and they would eat at like 3:00, 6:00 and 9:00, but it took them an hour to eat so by the time you got them back to sleep you could only get an hour of sleep yourself. I remember they came home the day after they were born and I was so worried -- David had missed quite a bit of work so he had to go in and I was afraid that because the boys were preemies they wouldn't wake up to eat, so I told David, "Call me at midnight because I'll fall asleep and I'll feel so terrible that I'm starving my babies." He said that he would and off he went to work.

The phone rang at about quarter to midnight and there in the background he could hear "Waaa! Wah! Wah!" They were LOUD! I heard his voice saying, "Annette, it's time to feed the babies." And I laughed, "Honey, I don't think that's gonna be a problem! They *know* when they want to eat. We'll *never* have to wake them up!"

CHAPTER SIX

"On to Greener Pastures -- if they let us"

It's funny the things we take for granted about our bodies. I remember after the mastectomy I woke up and was very aware of my breathing. I noticed that my chest didn't heave up and down as I inhaled and exhaled. There was just nothing there. It was empty. I gingerly touched my chest, feeling around and I could tell my breast was gone, leaving just an indentation where it had been. The skin had been pulled smooth, like the chest of a ten-year-old but there wasn't even a nipple there. It was very strange. The pain however, was quite mild compared to that of my first surgery. I was in the surgical ward this time instead of maternity. We had a really big beautiful room that had a television, VCR and a couch. David stayed with me the whole three days. We'd get videos from the front desk and watch movies all day long. We ordered guest trays for him so we could eat together. We had like a three day "date" and actually had a good time!

David was sitting by my bed reading the newspaper when he said, "Guess what, Annette, there's a piece of land out in Herriman that's only $16,500."

By now we'd sold our house and already picked out the house we wanted to build. We just needed land to build on but everything we'd looked at was out of our price range. I agreed we should see this land in Herriman sometime.

The next day I got discharged from the hospital, and instead of taking me home David drove me clear out to Herriman (about 30 minutes away) to inspect this piece of property! I felt so sick, I wanted to just say, "Take me *home*!" But I knew this was important to him.

When we finally got out there I stood on the lot and had the feeling we were *supposed* to be there. "David," I said, "This is supposed to be our land. I just know it."

"Are you sure?" he asked. "You know I don't get a feeling about this kind of stuff."

I looked around again, stared up at the sky and the beautiful mountains off in the distance and said, "Yeah.... this is it. I think we should talk to our realtor right now and have her make an offer."

I called her and she tried to talk me out of it.

"On to Greener Pastures--if they let us"

"Oh Annette, you don't want to live way out in Herriman," she protested.

"But we saw the lot and it's perfect. We really want it." I said.

"But Herriman is so far from everything. Do you realize all the driving you'll have to do? How far you'll have to go to get groceries? Not to mention doctor appointments and the medical treatments you'll be facing!"

"David and I have discussed those things and we *still* really want this land. Please call and give them our offer."

"Before I do that, I'd like to take a look at it myself. I'll go out this afternoon and get back to you."

The realtor called me back a few hours later and her attitude had changed 180 degrees. "Annette, you're right. We have to get you that lot. It's really much nicer than I expected," she conceded.

We made an offer on the land but it was rejected. So we said, "Okay, we'll give them the asking price," because we knew this was supposed to be for us. Well, the owners got a little strange on us and tried to take us for a ride. They wanted us to sign a contract saying we'd give them $5000 down and then if THEY decided not to sell they could keep our money no matter what! The realtor told them about what we were going through with the cancer and twins and so on. She explained, "These kids cannot afford to lose that kind of money." She told them we would buy the land in six weeks, paid in cash and that our down payment would be in a secured account so no one could touch it. I feel like the only reason they agreed to our terms was because I was sick.

When we left our house in West Jordan -- the week I had my mastectomy -- we moved into a little -- and I do mean LITTLE, two bedroom twin home that my mom and step-dad owned. We were cramped but we were able to live there rent free which allowed us to save up the money we needed. My mom was the Relief Society president in her ward at the time so a lot of people helped us out with meals and taking care of my family. My children had to be shifted around from home to home to be cared for. I didn't like that, even though it was necessary. I just felt so bad that I never really got to be a mother to my twins when they were babies. But luckily the kids didn't seem to mind. They appeared to have a good time. I know the boys were spoiled rotten.

CHAPTER SEVEN

"Tips for the Chemo Diet"

After we had looked at the land in Herriman I came home and fell into bed exhausted. Five hours later I woke up feeling terrible. I kept shivering. "David, I'm freezing."

He put a comforter over me and felt my forehead. "You're burning up!" He rummaged around for a thermometer and finally located one. After taking my temperature he announced, "It's 105.8 degrees. You're sick!"

No kidding. I felt horrible. My whole body ached. I had chills and my clothes were damp from perspiration. "David, I want a blessing."

"Ok, I'll call the bishop," he promised.

A few minutes later the bishop and a neighbor arrived at our door to give me a priesthood blessing. They anointed me with consecrated oil then laid their hands upon my head and blessed me that I would recover. When they were done the bishop looked at me and commented, "Gosh, Annette, when I first got here you looked like death. It's nice to see some color coming back into your face."

We called Dr. Jack and he prescribed an antibiotic for me since he was sure I had developed an infection. David ran to get that and some Tylenol.

Three days later I went to the doctor to get my stitches out. He looked at the wound and said, "Hmm... just a minute." I wasn't looking at what he was doing because I couldn't stand to watch. But my mom was there and she said he took a scalpel and cut me back open -- I didn't feel it because I didn't have any feeling there after they cut all the nerves. He drained out half a cup of black ooze which was the infection. It was so disgusting. After that I had a big gaping hole in my chest. I could even see the muscle through it.

I decided to play a joke on my aunt Sherrie who is known to gag easily. The next time I saw her I called out "Hey Aunt Sherrie, come look at this!" When she came over I pulled my shirt aside and showed her the big hole in my chest. She took one look and almost threw up! I think she was the only person I showed it to. She had been so wonderful taking me to chemo, watching my kids, running me everywhere. And this is how I repaid her! She may not have appreciated my sense of humor but she loved me anyway.

I'd had my mastectomy on January 17, 1992. Dr. Legant wanted me to start on chemo right away but she decided it was better for me to wait until I'd healed from the surgery and the infection was gone. I was dreading chemo because I knew I'd lose my hair. I became obsessed over losing it. That is all I worried about. It didn't matter to me that I might throw up or feel tired or have chemicals in my body. I was just freaking out that I was going to lose my hair.

I tried to buy myself a little more time. At my February 24th appointment I mentioned to the doctor somewhat hopefully, "Um... you know... my twins are being blessed in church on March 1st, so why don't we wait one more week so that I can still have my hair for that?" I did not want to be bald when all my friends and family came to the blessing.

But Dr. Legant told me, "You won't lose your hair for at least a couple weeks, so you should be fine."

I was crestfallen. "You mean I really have to start chemo now?"

She was firm in her reply, "Yes. We've waited as long as we can."

I was really nervous about what chemo would feel like. I had a friend with a brain tumor and she told me that they gave her chemo with something in it that stung really bad as it went into her arm. I kept thinking chemo was going to kill me. I didn't want more pain.

Well, let me just say that chemo really wasn't as bad as I expected it to be. It was no picnic either. The needles were irritating. After a couple sets of chemo my veins were basically worthless. They collapsed easily and I'd have to be stuck and poked several times to get the needle in. I couldn't feel the chemo going into me but I would get sick to my stomach. They have wonderful anti-nausea stuff though that they put in with the chemo and it made me feel really out of it. It was actually kind of nice. It was definitely better than throwing up.

As I went through this experience I learned a few tricks. I had to learn one the hard way. As I prepared for my first set of chemo I thought, "I won't eat and that way there won't be anything to throw up." So I took chemo on an empty stomach. Big mistake. When I got home I was hungry so I ate something and then went to sleep. At about 7:00 pm that night I woke up and started heaving my guts out. I was *so sick*. I threw up and threw up. It was awful because it was very acidic from the chemicals so it burned my esophagus and throat as it came up. After that I learned to eat FIRST so the chemo wouldn't hit an empty stomach. It worked much better. I also learned that they usually give you a very high dose your first time to see how you are affected, and then they regulate it from there. I wish I had known all of this beforehand.

I also took pills every day as part of my chemotherapy. The pills made my gums bleed and gave me sores in my mouth. At my second set they cut the dosage way down so after that I didn't get very many sores in my mouth. My gums would bleed sometimes when I brushed my teeth but it wasn't too bad. I learned to deal with it. It sounds worse than it really is.

CHAPTER EIGHT

"Gotta Go, Gotta Go, Gotta Go Right Now"

Right after my first set of chemo, and before my hair fell out (I kept track of how things happened by remembering if I had hair or not!) I received a call from a lady in the "Mother of Twins" group. She offered to pick me up for one of their monthly meetings. I thought it sounded fun so I said I'd go. We went to St. Mark's hospital and about the middle of the meeting I suddenly felt very sick. I felt like I had the flu or something. I went out to the restroom and I had absolutely the *worst* case of diarrhea I'd ever had in my life! Every time I stood up I would get completely sick again and have to sit right back down. I sat there worrying, *What am I going to do? How am I going to make it home from here all the way back to West Valley without letting loose everywhere?*

I missed the rest of the meeting because I had to stay in the bathroom. I felt awful both physically and emotionally. I didn't know the ladies I had come with very well and I was so embarrassed to tell them what was happening. When the meeting let out they found me in the hall. One of them suggested we all go out for pie. I took a deep breath and said, "I am *really* sorry, but I have diarrhea like you wouldn't believe. I think this is how the chemo is affecting me." I asked them if they would mind running me home and they said that was fine. We got into the car and about halfway home I needed to stop at a

"Gotta Go, Gotta Go, Gotta Go Right Now"

Hardees restaurant to use the bathroom. We were almost to my house when I could feel it coming on again. *Oh please,* I prayed, *please help me to not get sick in this lady's car! I don't want to "lose it" all over her nice leather seats! Please help me make it home.*

The car pulled into my driveway and I didn't give them a second to chat. As soon as the car stopped I piled out, hastily mumbling my thanks and apologies. I closed the car door and at that moment my insides exploded --- everywhere. It was so disgusting! I am so glad it was dark outside so they didn't see or suspect anything.

I hurried inside to take a shower and change my clothes. I hadn't eaten anything all day and I was getting very dehydrated. I was scared. "David, please run to the store and get me some Sprite and Immodium." I begged. "I'm sooo sick."

He quickly returned with it and it helped me a little. I felt the urge to go again but didn't make it to the bathroom and found myself taking another shower and having David throw in another load of laundry.

"Annette, are you going to be okay?" David asked worriedly, "You've gone like five times in the last fifteen minutes."

"I think I'll be okay once the Immodium starts to work," I answered weakly. It proved to be true.

At my next oncology appointment I told my doctor how badly it affected my intestines. She didn't think it was related to the chemo. I did because I'd read how chemo kills fast growing cells and that is what we have in our intestines. She argued that chemo usually didn't cause diarrhea in the proportions I'd had. She said to watch and see what happened. So I did. And guess what? After every set of chemo it

"Gotta Go, Gotta Go, Gotta Go Right Now" happened. But not as bad as that first time. Still, I learned to plan my schedule so I would stay home a certain number of days after each treatment.

At my second set of chemo they cut the dosage down quite a bit, but they also cut way back on the anti-nausea medication so I threw up a lot that time. I think I lost four pounds that week. I just couldn't keep anything down. I probably could have thrown up every day but I fought it really hard because it burned so badly coming up. I lived on a couple of pieces of toast a day since that was all I could eat. I didn't take the anti nausea pills they gave me because they made me feel weird. I just relied on the anti nausea they would put in the chemo IV. I begged them to give me extra. They did and it worked really well. I'd sleep about two days.

CHAPTER NINE

"I Want My Chemo and I Want it NOW!"

Just when I was getting the routine down for my weeks on and off chemo I got another curve ball thrown at me. Angie came home from school one day all upset.

"Mom, I have spots," she cried.

"What do you mean?" I asked. "Come here and let me look." She pointed to one spot and then another. I recognized them. I'd had hundreds of them myself when I was twelve.

"I Want My Chemo and I Want it NOW!"

"Oh Angie," I moaned, "You've got chicken pox."

She had a mild case -- probably a total of 42 on her whole body. She was so paranoid about getting scars that she was very careful not to pick at them. Soon Jessica came down with them and she had about 42 just in her armpit! She had them *everywhere*. She also thought it was great fun to pick them off. Then it wasn't long before both boys broke out and to make matters worse, the twins also had ear infections! For the most part I took care of all these sick kids *by myself.* David was working and on evenings and weekends he had to help build our house in Herriman. I felt so guilty about needing help when I was chemo that I couldn't bring myself to ask for help now. When I did mention it to a couple of people their reaction was "Oh, my kids haven't had chicken pox yet and I don't want them to get it." So I just dealt with it. All four kids kept me up every night. The boys were the worst because of the ear infections. I was not getting any sleep. In desperation I called my sister-in-law Susan and begged her to come over. I'd only had three hours of sleep in three days. I was having a nervous breakdown.

She came over, took care of the kids *and* cleaned my house while I caught up on my sleep. I was so thankful. It wasn't until much later that I learned I could have *died* from my kids having chicken pox because my immune system was compromised from the chemo. I am lucky nothing happened from that! Blessings in disguise!

A day or so later it was time for chemo again. This meant I'd get a nice vacation because I'd sleep for a couple days and the kids would be at other people's houses. I walked into the hospital actually smiling. I was *so* excited!

"I Want My Chemo and I Want it NOW!"

"Well, you're sure happy today," one of the nurses commented.

"I get to have chemo today! Yay!" I grinned.

She looked at me like I was crazy. After the blood was drawn I glanced through a magazine as I waited for them to call me back for my treatment.

"Oh Annette," one of the nurses reported, "we can't give you your chemo today. Your white cell count is too low."

I burst out bawling and begged, "Please! Can't you just give it to me anyway??"

Another nurse had heard our conversation and came over to check on me. "What's wrong?" she asked.

"I want my chemo!" I demanded.

The nurses looked at each other in shock and one of them laughed, "Gosh Annette, we've *never* had anybody *beg* for chemo before!"

I wiped the tears away and sniffed, "You've never had anybody with four kids who have had chicken pox and ear infections so she hasn't slept for days before!"

The nurses sympathized but stood firm, "Well, we're sorry, but we can't give it to you. Come back in about ten days."

By the time I could receive my next set it had been a total of five weeks since Angie got chicken pox. I'd gone through all of that time with hardly any sleep. No wonder my white cell count was low! The whole ordeal was something I didn't think I'd live through. Sleep deprivation is an awful thing. New moms get it anyway --- new moms with twins get it twice as bad. But a new mom with newborn twins, kids with chickenpox and cancer really ranks high on the "I'm about ready to lose it" scale.

CHAPTER TEN

"No More Tangles"

Speaking of losing things, let's talk about my hair. I had long, blonde hair. I liked my hair. My husband liked my hair. Hair was important to me --- after all, I was a beautician. People would suggest that I just cut it all off since I was going to lose it anyway.

My response to that was --- NO way! Not on your life! I would tell people, "If God can move mountains; He can keep hair on my head." I was determined to just have the faith that He could. I was a cocky thing wasn't I -- daring God? It's not something I recommend. But I felt like I deserved it. I'd had my breast cut off; I'd had to endure the pain of surgery. I'd had to suffer through chemotherapy -- but I just didn't have to agree to cut my hair off!

My doctor told me about a program sponsored by the American Cancer Society called "Reach to Recovery." They have women volunteers who are breast cancer survivors that come to your home to visit after you've been diagnosed. A lady from the program came out to talk to me. She'd had breast cancer and gone through chemo so we talked about that. I was dying to ask about the hair thing.

"What was it like when your hair fell out?" I asked.

"Oh, mine didn't fall out because I had a different kind of chemo than yours," she replied.

"Well, do you know when I can expect mine to fall out?"

"From what I've been told, it should go in about two weeks."

Two weeks later I still had all my hair. She happened to call me up one afternoon. "Is your hair falling out?" she asked.

"Nope," I replied.

"Wow!" she exclaimed impressed, "that's incredible. I've asked around and *everybody's* hair is usually falling out by now."

I felt really good about that and I figured I had enough faith to keep my hair for three or four more days.

And I did.

But then it started to fall out a little at a time when I brushed it. After about four days my part was getting kind of wide so it was time to cover it. I tried a hat, but it didn't look good on me. I went out and bought a wig. I hated it. I thought

I'd never wear it because I felt like a dork in it. But once I got used to it I realized it looked pretty good. In fact a lot of people didn't even know it was a wig. People who hadn't seen me for awhile just thought I'd done something different to my hair. The only ones who could tell right off were my friends who were also beauticians.

Looking back I realize how odd I acted about losing my hair. I literally planned my life around it. For example, one day a friend called to invite me to lunch.

I looked at my calendar and said, "Ok... if my hair hasn't fallen out by Tuesday then we can do lunch." And that is really how it was --I had to "schedule" everything around it.

One of my clients had recently been diagnosed with breast cancer and had a mastectomy. She came over for a haircut one day. I had just washed my own hair before she arrived and I had it pulled back in a braid. As I started cutting her hair I felt a strange sensation on the back of my head. It felt like something had pulled loose. It suddenly dawned on me what had happened and I cried out, "Oh my gosh, I think my hair just fell out!"

She tried to calm me down. "It's okay, Annette. Why don't you comb it out right now while I'm here? Let me see it."

I had already combed out a little garbage can full upstairs when I had washed it. I pulled the elastic off the end of the braid and ran my fingers through to loosen it. I picked up my comb and ran it through my hair. *Handfuls* came out. Fallen strands covered my shoulders, cascaded down the front and back of me and collected in a pile on the floor at my feet. I felt weak in the knees.

"Oh my goodness Annette," she kept saying over and over. The more that came out, the more she would repeat it. I have a lot of hair, so even though tons came out, I still had quite a bit left on my head. I wasn't bald or anything -- yet.

I saw the doctor on a Thursday and I wore a hat because I still had a few bangs left. But on Friday I had to wear the wig because it was pretty much all gone. When I looked in a mirror I thought I looked like a little old man. That sure wasn't a good boost for my self esteem! I had about 20 hairs that never fell out. I left them there. I couldn't bear to cut them off either.

Ok... I admit that it was a lot nicer to just have the hair gone and not worry about having it go. I really wasted a lot of time and energy on that. I even called people that I knew who had cancer -- but none of them had lost their hair --- and I'd bug them for any information they could give me. "Tell me how is my hair going to fall out?"

The usual reply was, "In clumps."

That wasn't good enough for me. I wanted more specific information.

"Okay," I'd say exasperated, "am I going to be standing in the middle of the mall one day and my hair just falls off in a clump and I am standing there bald?" Nobody knew for sure so I *still* didn't know what to expect. I wanted to be totally prepared for it. I was even willing to stay home and not leave for fear it would fall off in public!

As it turned out, it fell out a little at a time.... usually when I was brushing it. Because I braided it in the back, the hair that would fall out during the day would just stay in the braid and come out when I combed it. I now *understand* why people opt to cut their hair short or shave their head. But that wasn't an option I was willing to use at that time.

It was after I had survived this major catastrophe -- losing my hair --- that I adopted a new attitude. Well, maybe it was an attitude I'd always had, but I really used it now. I called it my "whatever" attitude. I used it to deal with everything that happened each day. I let it all roll off my back. I took life just one hour at a time. I tried to stop worrying about the future or the "what if's." As you've come to realize through reading this book --- I am a person who worries and has to know everything that has, or will happen. But now, no matter what came at me I shrugged my shoulders and said, "Whatever." And that is how I survived.

I also spent a lot of time analyzing why Heavenly Father let this happen to me. I wanted to raise my children. I didn't want anyone else to raise them. I needed to be their mother. I needed to give them love, and teach them how to grow up to be good people. But the more I thought that everything would turn out alright... the more uneasy I felt deep down inside that maybe things were *not* going to end up the way I hoped.

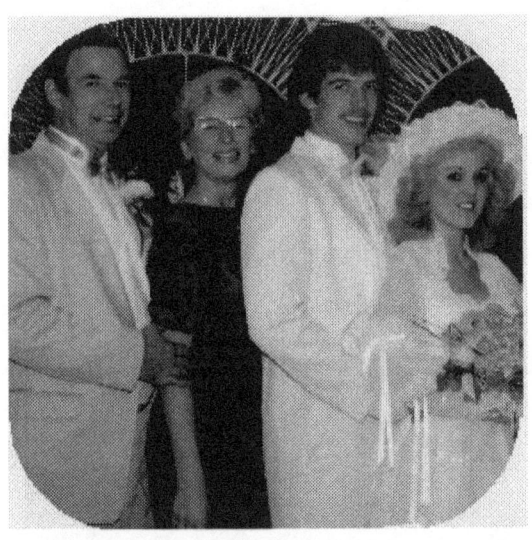

Just like any couple starting out in life... we had no idea what lay ahead. This was our wedding day, November 20, 1984 with David's mom and dad.

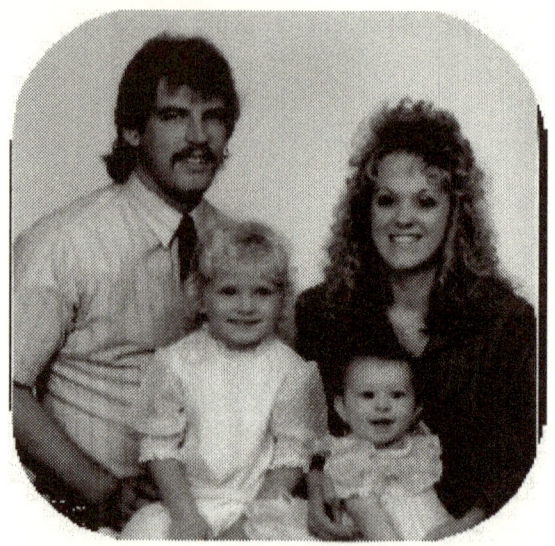

A family photo when Angie and Jessica were little

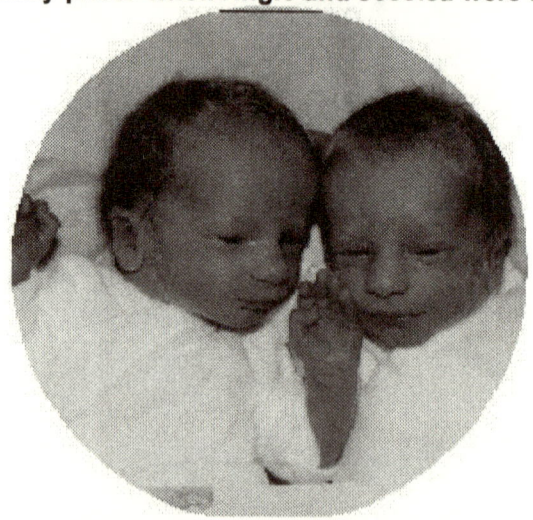

TWINS! Scott and Shane arrived Dec. 28, 1991. I had them naturally, no anesthetic – and was the talk of the maternity ward!

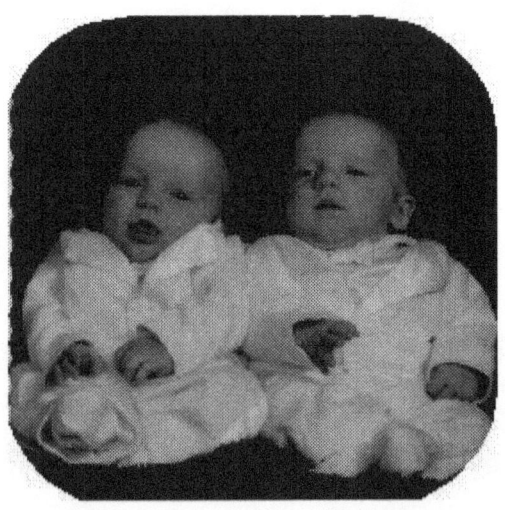

The boys were blessed in the ward in West Jordan where they were born. I had just started chemotherapy.

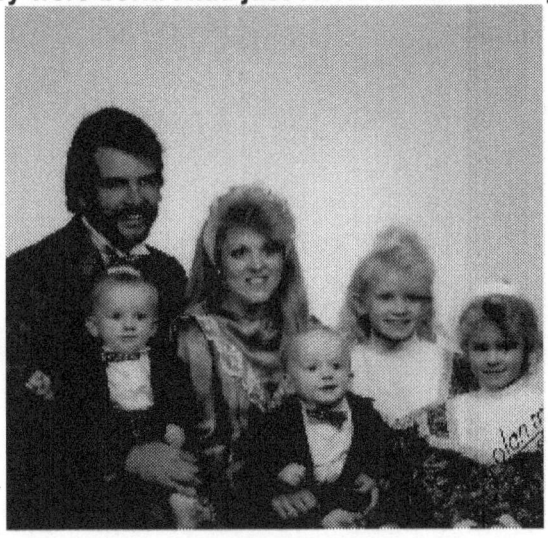

I was going through chemo and had to wear a wig for this picture.

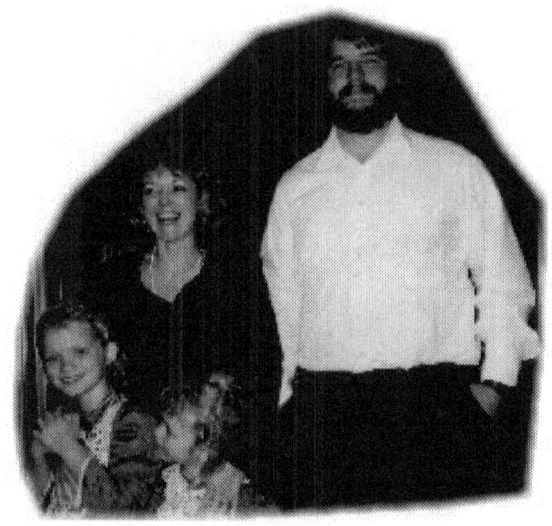

At Angie's baptism I had my own hair again, but it was shorter than I like it.

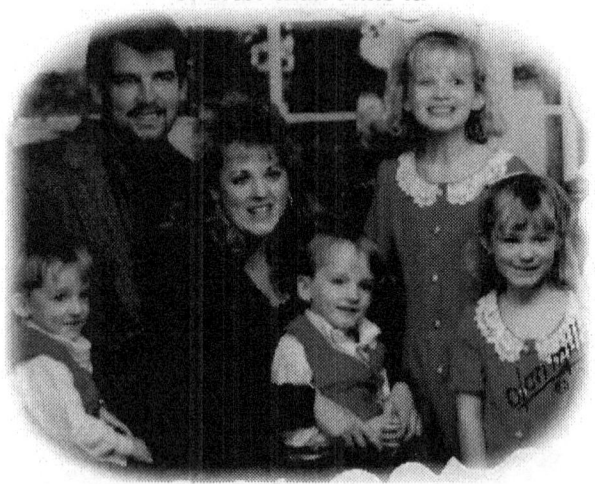

We did this family photo in 1994 for Christmas and all of my hair was back!

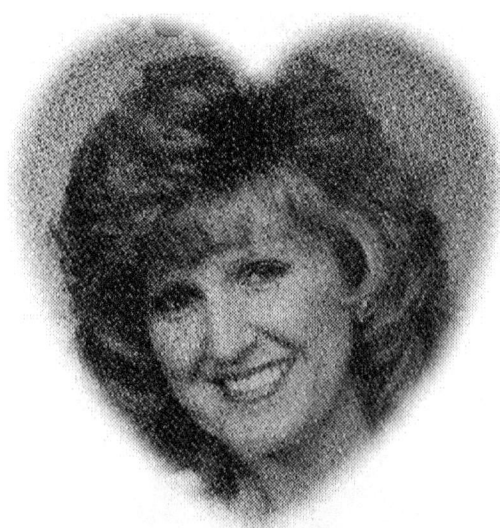

This is Joslyn. We became the best of friends as we fought together against breast cancer. Joselyn lost her fight in May of 1997.

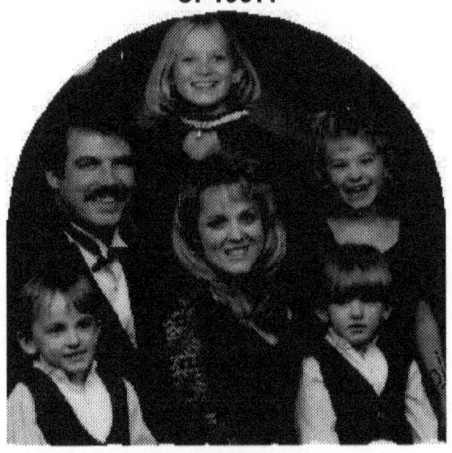

This photo was taken at my brother Shane's wedding. I didn't find out until a couple of months later that I had 11 brain tumors.

There's Always a Rainbow

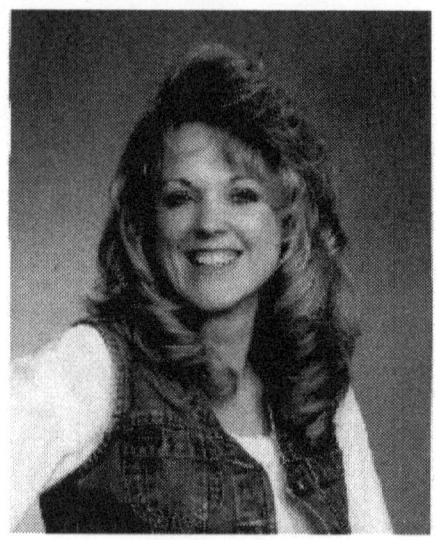

I had this photo done when I thought I had beat the cancer
for good, and all my hair had grown back. But a little voice
inside me told me it was going to be my obituary photo...
and it was.

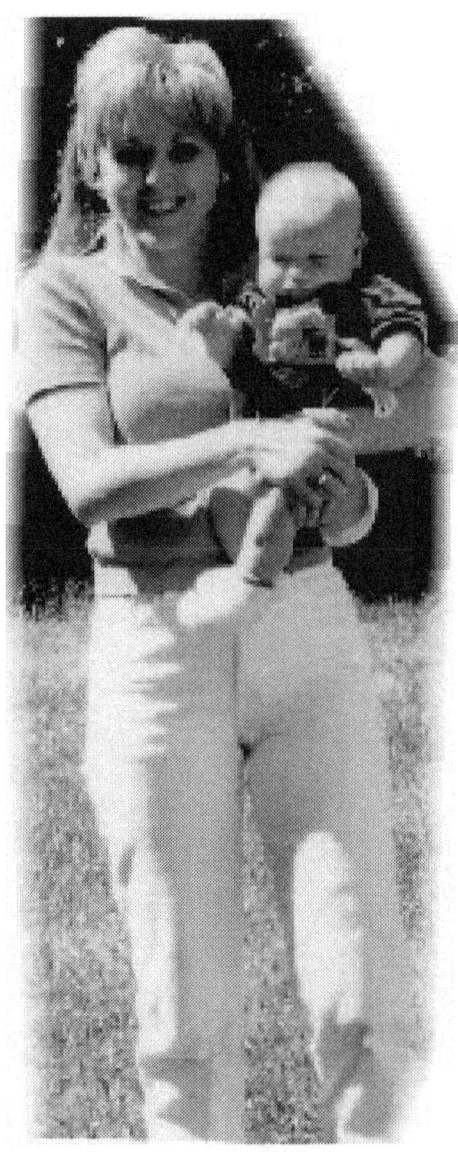

**Memorial Day, 1997 with my nephew Colton. I had lost my
hair to radiation and had to buy another wig.**

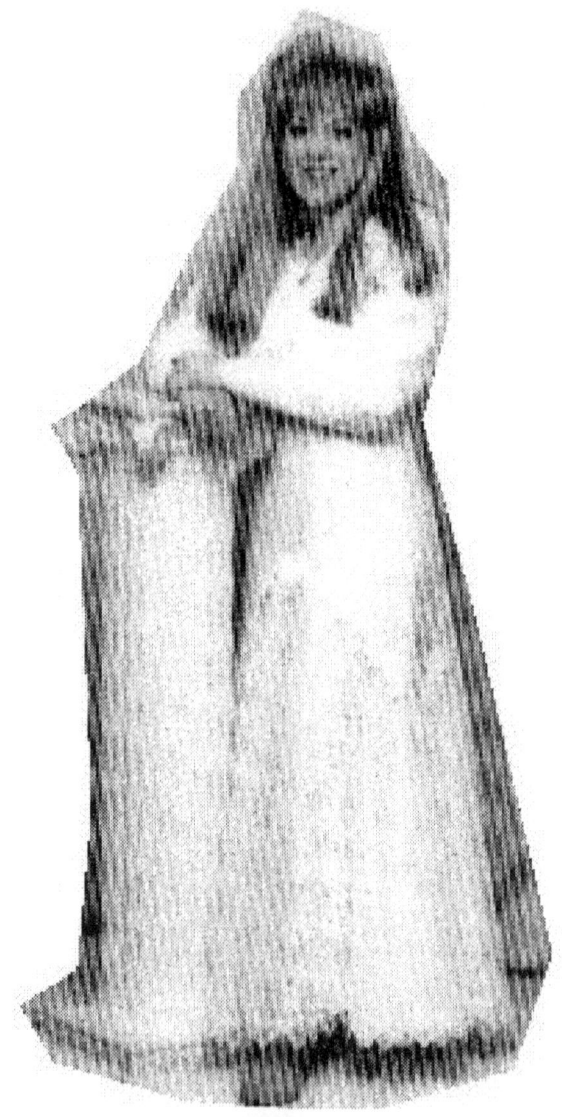

My mom made this dress for me to be buried in. I had a
photo taken in it because I wanted her to have it. I thought it
was the prettiest dress she ever made.

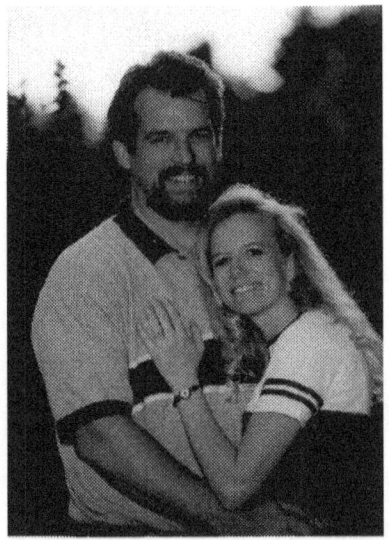

David and Sheri find happiness together.

CHAPTER ELEVEN
"I Can't Believe I Ate The Whole Thing!"

We were still living in my mom's twin home when it came time to bless the twins. I felt it was necessary to bless them in our West Jordan ward -- the one where they had been born. At the blessing I got up to bear my testimony. I remember saying: "I know Heavenly Father doesn't give us tests that we can't handle... but I'm sure he's mixed me up with somebody else." I thanked the ward for the dinners and the baby-sitting. They had really gone way above and beyond the call of duty to help us. I felt like I could never thank them enough. My boys were the ward's babies too. They had even given me a beautiful baby shower because I didn't have any boy things. I'm so glad we were able to bless them there.

The Lord blessed us in ways we couldn't even see at the time. We had so many medical bills --- we were really strapped financially. We had to come up with $10,000 for our house. We got $3000 from the sale of our West Jordan home so that meant we somehow had to come up with another $7000. I don't know how we did it but by the time we moved into our new home we had paid off the babies' hospital bill and most of the other medical bills *and* we had the money for closing costs. I have no clue how we did that except the Lord had to have opened the windows of heaven.

At the end of June I was more than halfway through the chemo. I had two more sets to go. I went in for the fifth set and was told that my immune system was again too low so I couldn't have it. I was ticked.

"Well, that's really going to mess up my schedule because my mother and father-in-law are coming to town and I have to be moved into my new house. Can't you just give it to me anyway?"

The nurse folded her arms, looked at me sternly and said, "Annette! When we tell you, you can't have chemo *then you can't have it!*"

So I waited another week.

David's mom and dad came out and helped us move into our new house. I was really ticked off that I had to do chemo while they were here. I was determined not to miss out on any of the fun while they were in town. I had chemo on Monday. On Tuesday the family decided to get together for lunch at TGIFridays. David couldn't go so I brought Angie with me. I looked at the menu and decided I just HAD to have the chimichanga! I don't know why but it sounded sooo good to me.

Everyone was shocked and kept saying, "Annette! You just had chemo and you want to eat a *chimichanga*? Are you *crazy*?"

Can you believe I ate the *whole* thing? I ate everything on my plate and I usually don't do that even when I'm well! But it tasted sooo good. It was the best chimichanga I ever ate. But as luck would have it, my body rejected it and a few hours later I got sick. It lasted for three days. Every time I threw up or had diarrhea David would say "I can't believe you did that. Was it really worth it?"

And I'd say, "Yup! It *was* worth it!"

Finally the countdown was over. I was going to the hospital for what would be my very last set of chemo. No more needles. No more nausea.

I thought I'd be so excited to have it over that it wouldn't even bother me.

I was wrong.

I saw the needle and my stomach retched. "Hand me the garbage can, I'm going to throw up!" I yelled at the nurse.

"But we haven't even given it to you yet!" she chuckled.

I moaned, "I don't care! I'm sick!" Actually I didn't get sick but I thought I would. It was horrible to the end. They would often have to stick me seven or eight times to find a vein. The damage it did to me psychologically was even worse. I couldn't look at a sewing needle for TWO YEARS without wanting to throw up.

CHAPTER TWELVE

"Tip-toe through Radiation"

The summer day was hot as I sat in Dr. Legant's office waiting to hear what my next step in treatment would be.

"You've made it through surgery and chemo," she began, "but we're not finished yet. I'd like you to go for twenty-five radiation treatments."

Twenty-five! I gasped, wondering how many months that would take.

"You need to come in five times a week, for five weeks," she explained. "When do you want to start?"

"As soon as possible -- let's just get it over with," I sighed.

I went in the very next day to be marked for the areas they would be radiating. Talk about a strange experience! It's an odd feeling to see lines and dots drawn on your body. For the next month or so most of my days revolved around radiation. It was a thirty minute drive each way from Herriman to Murray. Most of the time, I also had to run my kids to a babysitter and go pick them up again.

Every time I went in for a treatment the radiologist would say "Oh Annette, I'm so sorry we have to do this to you."

I'd respond, "Please! This is a *picnic* compared to chemo!"

It may have been easier, but to me it was much *scarier* to get radiation. With chemo I saw the needle, I saw the tubes, I saw the bag of chemicals. I was aware of what was happening. But with radiation I was put into a room with 7 foot thick lead walls. I laid on a cold table. The door would shut and I would be left completely alone. I couldn't see what was happening. I wanted to call out, "Wait! Come back here! Don't leave me here all by myself!" (Yes, I realize I have a problem with being left alone.) The actual treatment itself was nothing. I thought I'd feel heat or something but I felt nothing at all. I would lay there wondering if it was done or not because I couldn't even tell.

My grandpa died while I was going through the radiation treatments. I didn't go to his funeral because it was at the same time as a treatment and I didn't know that it would have been okay for me to miss one. I found out later that I could have gone without it causing a problem. I didn't think to ask anyone about it at the time. I felt kind of bad about missing the funeral, but maybe it was a good thing because emotionally I wasn't able to handle seeing death. Just sitting in the waiting room to get chemo or radiation I would be surrounded by so many people with cancer.... and I knew that most of them were going to die. I met a lot of really nice people and it was so sad to think that many of them would not be cured despite everything they did.

It was during this time that I got a phone call from a girl recently diagnosed with breast cancer. I'm not sure if my doctor gave her my number or what but she wanted to talk to me because she was going through the same type of chemo that I had. We talked on the phone for a long time.

"I'd love to meet you Annette. You have such a positive attitude. I really like that. Would you mind meeting me in person?" she asked.

"Sure," I told her, "I'm going in tomorrow for my last radiation treatment. Why don't you just meet me at the hospital? Then you can sort of see what it's like in case you have to go through it too."

We met in the hospital cafeteria to talk. I found out she had four children but was not married. She had a live-in boyfriend who wasn't real supportive.

I felt prompted to ask her, "So what do you believe? Are you religious at all?"

"No," she replied, "I'm an atheist. I don't believe in God. I don't really care much for religion. It's too restrictive."

I felt bad for her that she didn't have the peace that faith can bring. "I guess it's hard for you to find any purpose to what you're going through then." I commented.

"What do you mean by that?" she queried.

I shifted my position in the chair, "Well... I believe that we're sent here to be tried and tested in all things. So for me... having cancer is a test. When I pray, I receive help and comfort and strength to deal with everything I'm going through. But I guess you wouldn't pray because you don't believe anyone is there." I paused to see how she was responding to this because I didn't want to offend her; she was listening intently. I continued, "To me it would be a really horrible thing to be diagnosed with cancer and not believe in any purpose for it. People die from cancer and if I thought that I just ceased to exist when I die then that would cause me a lot of despair. I want to live --- but I'm not *afraid* of death because of what I believe."

She shook her head and snorted, "I don't think I can find a purpose for this---" she pointed to her flat chest and bald head.

As we continued talking I could see she *was* searching for something to help her cope. We handled the same situation so differently.

"So how come you look so good?" she asked, changing the subject.

The differences in our appearance were strikingly opposite. I was dressed nicely and had on a wig and makeup. She wore no make-up, baggy clothes, and a hat that didn't cover her baldness very well. She looked like the stereotypical cancer patient. I wanted her to know that she could look good too if she cared enough about herself. "I just refuse to look like a cancer patient," I shrugged. "You might be sick," I continued, "but the whole world doesn't have to know. I feel like if I look awful then I am letting the cancer win. I'd rather fight back with everything I've got."

She wanted to see my scar so I went ahead and showed it to her. She showed me hers. I know you might think that is an odd thing for two strangers to do but I felt like that area of my body wasn't really private anymore. There was no breast there -- there was basically *nothing* there so it didn't feel immodest. It was not a big deal. Her scar was really horrible. Whoever did her surgery did a terrible job. I felt so bad for her to be scarred like that. She had no interest in having reconstruction. It wasn't important to her.

With radiation finished it was time to visit my surgeon again because our medical insurance was covering everything 100 percent now. With this in mind I wanted to start reconstruction. I went in early October.

"It looks like we'll have to wait awhile to begin this," the doctor said. "The radiation burned you too badly and if we try to insert the expander it will rip your skin to shreds."

"How long is that going to take to heal?" I asked.

"Well, we'll give you some cream to rub on it which should speed up the healing process. See, there is a slight tear right here under your arm. That's going to have to heal up also. Come back in a few months and we'll look at it again."

A few *months*?

Six weeks later I went back. The nurse looked at me and asked, "Have you even had radiation yet?"

"Yeah," I answered, "Remember I was burned too much? That's why I had to come back."

"I can't even tell you ever had radiation! That's incredible!" she was stunned.

The doctor came in and asked me, "Tell me again how long it's been since you had radiation?"

"About two months," I answered.

"That's amazing. I have patients who are stilled burned after *four* months."

Well, I thought, *Heavenly Father knew I had a deadline with the insurance so He kindly speeded things up a bit!*

And for that, I was *very* grateful.

CHAPTER THIRTEEN

"Laughter, Tears and Reconstruction"

Let's have a moment of comic relief shall we? I just have to share with you one of the most embarrassing moments of my life which occurred around this time. I used to play the guitar and sing the song, "I'll Build You a Rainbow." It's a song about a little boy whose mother dies. As the ambulance drives away with her body his dad stands in the driveway crying. The boy looks up and right over their house is a rainbow. It's a very emotional song that is very important to me and close to my heart. My girls and I were invited to perform this song in a church sacrament meeting. We practiced it over and over at home. The girls knew the words by heart. But kids, as we all know.... can be unpredictable.

Sunday dawned bright and early as our moment in the spotlight arrived. I asked one of the young women to keep an eye on the twins out in the foyer so they wouldn't be distracting. The girls and I walked up to the stand and positioned ourselves with Angie on one side of me and Jessica on the other. I took my guitar out of the case, strummed the chords and began singing:

"I'll build you a rainbow, way up high above
Send down a sunbeam, plum full of love
Sprinkle down raindrops, tear drops of joy
I'll be happy as springtime watching over my
boy...."

Out of the corner of my eye I saw Scott running up and down one aisle and Shane climbing the chairs in the back row. I wondered, *Where's my sitter? Isn't she paying attention to them?* Right about that time Angie decided she didn't want to sing anymore so she started whispering in my ear. I tried to ignore her and continue the song but it's really difficult to sing when I'm hearing "Mom, I don't want to do this," over and over.

I forged ahead. The song contains narration as well as singing and I was trying to remember how the story went when Jessica waltzed down the steps to the rail beside the podium. She climbed up on it and started putting one foot in front of the other, arms outstretched as if on a balance beam. She teetered back and forth with each step she took. Suddenly she lost her balance and fell with a loud thud on the floor and started crying.

"Laughter, Tears and Reconstruction"

I kept trying to sing:

"I'll build you a rainbow..."

Jessica climbed back on the rail to begin another gymnastic routine and everyone in the congregation was trying so hard not to laugh. I finally couldn't stand it. I stopped playing right in the middle of the song, pointed my finger at someone on the front row and said, "Could you get her down please?"

Then I turned to Angie and through my clenched teeth said "Just let me get through this okay?"

I finished the song, threw my guitar in the case, grabbed all of the kids and went directly home!

"How'd your song go?" David asked later that afternoon.

"Well," I chuckled, "it's something everyone will be talking about for a LONG time!"

What a disaster! That was supposed to be a spiritual song and it turned into a circus. Over time I've come to appreciate the humor in it. That was one sacrament musical number that went down in history for sure!

I finally decided that I was ready to face reconstruction. *This should be a piece of cake. The worst is all behind me.* Or so I thought. I soon learned reconstruction would be one of the most excruciating, painful things I've ever done. The pain was as intense as that of my first surgery when they had removed my lymph nodes.

A silicone implant was also inserted into my *right* breast so it would match the left after the reconstruction. (I didn't want to be "perky" on just one side.) In the left side they placed an expander which is an implant that they fill with fluid very slowly over several weeks to gradually stretch the skin. But the expander went in the same place where I'd had that awful infection. So what had happened is the muscle had grown into that space and adhered to the skin. I had to be cut through to the middle of the muscle to put in the implant. Maybe if that hadn't happened it wouldn't have been so bad. I would never discourage anyone from having reconstruction. It really does help you to feel whole again and improves your self esteem a lot.

When I woke up from that surgery pain emanated from my chest and coursed throughout my body like a recurring shock wave. I could not feed myself, go to the bathroom or walk. I was helpless. I think I should have stayed in the hospital for a couple of days, but I was told this was outpatient surgery and they sent me home.

The pain became crippling. Percodan barely numbed it to a point where I could *almost* tolerate it but not quite. I was suffering. If I tried to move, my body buckled from the agony. I had no strength to fight anymore. I just wanted to go to sleep and not deal with it. The boys were old enough to climb all over me now and it seemed that several times a day I was getting bumped, hit, smashed or used as a pillow right where the expander was.

Why did I do this? I agonized.

Six months later they removed the expander and inserted a saline implant. I wasn't even going to consider using a silicone one after all the horror stories in the news about how they leak and cause cancer. The last thing I needed was to purposely put something in my body that could cause cancer! I've had enough, thank you.

I expected this second operation to be as bad as the previous one, but it wasn't. I guess second surgeries are the lucky ones for me. I was able to sit up all by myself right after the operation! I was surprised at how easy it was. I was relieved that this recuperation would be easier. Maybe *now* I could start living a normal life again?

CHAPTER FOURTEEN

"Beginning the Crusade"

Looking back over the previous eighteen months I could tell I had changed a lot inside as well as out. My testimony of the gospel had grown and my relationship with my Heavenly Father had become *very* personal. There were times when I had truly felt His presence with me. I'd been given a taste of what Gethsemane was like for Jesus. He'd suffered both body and spirit -- so had I. He asked if it might be taken from him -- so had I. He resigned himself to his Father's will -- and so had I. I came to appreciate the tremendous sacrifice He made. I suffered only for myself. He suffered for all of us.

After my two reconstructive surgeries I got a call from a girl I had grown up with in West Valley. She knew of a lady in her ward who had just been diagnosed with breast cancer and she wanted me to call and talk to her since I'd been through it. She told me her name was Joslyn.

I called Joslyn right away. When I heard her voice a warm, tingling feeling came over me. It was like I already knew her. We hit it off instantly. We talked about all the different types of chemo and I tried to answer all of her questions. I learned she was the mother of five children -- her youngest was just three years old. We quickly became the best of friends.

One day Joslyn called me to ask for my help. "I want to go talk about breast cancer to the people at the American Cancer Society to see what is being done in researching this disease. I want you to come with me. Will you?"

I told her I would, so off we went. Joslyn was introduced at the meeting and she got up to give her speech. The lady sitting beside me leaned over and asked, "Are you her sister here to lend moral support?"

"No," I replied, "I'm also a breast cancer survivor."

Her jaw dropped a mile and she gasped, "No way! How old are you?"

I was now 29 years old. I told her a bit about my story and she was completely flabbergasted. She told me that the Breast Cancer task force really needed people and asked if Joslyn and I would be interested. By then Joslyn had finished her speech and was listening to the tail end of the conversation. We both agreed it was something we'd like to do. Let me tell you,

Joslyn did a LOT. One of the neatest things that she did was write a video called "Get a Clue" which is shown at St. Mark's hospital.

One of the ladies on the task force was trying to obtain a bunch of signatures on petitions to be taken to Washington D.C. and presented to President Bill Clinton. She asked us to help circulate the petitions. Then we were asked if we'd go to Washington for the rally. It sounded great, but we learned the expense would come out of our own pockets. The cost would be around $700 each. I decided to ask for donations from people I knew and Joslyn got a couple of businesses to sponsor her. Before we knew it we were flying off to the nations' capital.

CHAPTER FIFTEEN

"Front Page News"

Upon boarding the plane, Joslyn and I found ourselves stuck in the middle seats. Joslyn gets terribly airsick. Right after the plane took off she ran to the bathroom and stayed in there the *entire* two and a half hour flight! The stewardess had to practically drag her out of it to sit down when the plane was landing! The seat beside me was empty so she sat down with her airsick bag. A few minutes later I looked over and poor Joslyn had the bag up to her face.

"Joslyn, are you throwing up?" I asked.

She nodded affirmatively.

"Wow, you do that so quietly no one would even notice!" I joked. I was amazed at how discreet she was. She didn't make noise or anything! She just sat their daintily throwing up!

"You'll have to show me how to do that sometime!" I teased.

We were busy in Washington going to meetings and parties with political officials. When we had time, we went on a few tours. We were half an hour late once getting to the tour bus and everyone was so mad at us! They kept harassing us and finally Joslyn turned around and grumbled, "Hey! Get over it and get a life!" They left us alone after that.

We went to a rally where there was an exhibit called "Faces of Breast Cancer." Each state featured one or two women who had died of the disease. It was really difficult to look at because so many of them were under the age of 30. Most had left little children behind. It was so depressing to see that. It hit me that these women died of the same disease *that I have.* It gave me a strange feeling -- almost like a premonition that my face would one day be among them.

"How awful it would be to leave your family behind," I commented to Joslyn.

"I know," she agreed, "but when it's your time then there's nothing you can do."

"Oh yeah?" I challenged, "Well let me tell you, they'll have to drag me through the veil kicking and screaming!"

We continued looking at the exhibit and suddenly someone called our names to go get our photo taken. We walked over to the steps and suddenly lots of people we didn't know started running over to take our pictures! I thought, "Gosh, they must really like us!"

Later on I asked somebody about it and she said, "Didn't you know that Susan Love was standing right behind you?"

I didn't even see her! So for a minute I thought I was really popular, but then my bubble got burst when I was told, "Naw... they didn't really want *your* picture, they wanted the woman standing behind you."

The next morning we went to tour the Holocaust Museum. The tour guide told us that to see everything takes over 25 hours. We wanted to see as much as we could so we hurried along. We were there for four hours and we practically ran through it! It was one place, however, that I wish I hadn't gone to see.

I had been so psyched up to take these petitions to the president. Then we saw the faces of all those women who had died of breast cancer and we realized it could be our face up there. Then we saw all the atrocities that took place against the Jews and our minds couldn't comprehend that much evil. I was feeling tremendous sadness as we walked through the museum. I got a taste of the hopeless feeling that people must have when they are diagnosed with cancer and have no religious beliefs. I saw pictures of the Jews whose children were ripped from their arms and sent off to the furnaces and gas chambers. The despair they must have felt because they had no knowledge that Jesus is the Messiah! They didn't know that families could be together forever. To them death was the end. I couldn't shake the sadness. It enshrouded me in a cloak of darkness.

We left the awesome bleakness of the museum and headed to the breast cancer rally. The mood there was one of joviality and it raised our spirits. We all wore sunshine yellow T-shirts. It was an impressive sight to see thousands of women in yellow marching and cheering. It was an incredibly uplifting contrast to the grayness we'd left behind at the museum. We bought yardsticks to carry our signs and while we were doing that a bunch of black men behind us started following me and Joslyn.

"Hey," one of them said to me, "we know you -- you're a soap opera star aren't you?"

"No, sorry, I'm not." I smiled.

"Yes you are! We've seen you on TV."

I insisted I wasn't but they wouldn't believe me. Joslyn and I laughed so hard we about busted a gut. Actually I was kind of flattered. They were so sure I was a television celebrity and nothing I said would change their minds. I don't even know WHO they thought I was.

There were a ton of TV cameras there to cover the event. We walked to the back lawn of the White House where we saw several celebrities. The Revlon models and Linda Lavin were there. Linda Ellerbee and Susan Love gave speeches. I was standing beside my friend Ann, also from Utah when a group of reporters stopped to talk to us. I think it was because Ann was marching bald so she kind of stuck out. They asked if they could take her picture for the Washington Post. I started teasing her that she always got her picture in the paper. The reporters told me I could get in the photo too. Sure enough, the next morning we were in the Washington Post. Utah had one of the biggest groups there of any state and I thought that was really neat.

We met with our state representatives and had the chance to talk to Senator Orrin Hatch and Karen Shepherd and Bob Bennett. They asked us to prepare a little talk to give in front of everybody. I didn't want to so I told Joslyn to do it. She talked to them but then somebody blurted out that I had been pregnant with twins when I was diagnosed. So then they wanted to hear from *me*. I gave a brief overview of all I'd been through and afterwards Senator Hatch approached me and said, "Gosh Annette, I need to give you a hug!" He gave me a great big hug and then posed for a photo with me and Joslyn. I really liked Senator Hatch. He's a very kind, caring and genuine man.

That night, after one of the busiest days of our lives, Joslyn became really ill because she was still on chemotherapy at the time and she was exhausted. She soon felt better and we were able to do more sight seeing. We saw a lot of homeless people. One day we were walking and saw a homeless black lady who had no teeth. Joslyn gave her all the change she had and a piece of pizza. It felt good to help someone, but sad that it didn't make much of a difference in the lady's situation. Washington

was nice, but a real culture shock for me.

CHAPTER SIXTEEN

"Magazines and Mischief"

After returning from Washington Joslyn asked me to be in the cancer video she was making. I thought it sounded like fun so I said yes. I met a lady there named Lillian Lee and we started talking. We'd both been diagnosed around the same time. She worked with another lady who wrote for different magazines. Lillian asked if she could tell this woman about me. I said sure.

The next thing I knew, I got a phone call asking for a magazine interview! I said okay and this gal wrote up a paragraph about me, submitted it to the magazine and then told me they had asked her to do a full feature story about me! I spent many hours on the phone with her and her editor. They sent a photographer out to my house. He shot several rolls of film of me and the family. The article was published in the September 13, 1994 issue of *Woman's World* magazine. It was kind of cool.

About a month later I was also featured in an article for our local Deseret News along with an artist named Matushka. She did some really abstract portraits of herself without a breast. I thought she was a little bit "out there" -- if you know what I mean.

I think the difference between Matushka and me is that she was all consumed with the physical part of breast cancer. She made paper mache models of her torso before she lost her breast and then did some awful pictures of herself with her mastectomy scar. She didn't have reconstruction or anything. I think she focused too much on the physical while I tried to approach my cancer experience from a spiritual perspective. I saw it as a test, a trial, something to go through, learn from, and overcome. She looked at it as being maimed for life and that it was a horrible, ugly thing that could never be changed. I felt like the physical wasn't the most important part. My belief is that one day I will be resurrected whole and well. I'll have my breast and my hair forever. While I'm here I can wear a wig -- my hair will grow back... I can have a new breast constructed.... so what is the big deal? I realized that we all look at the world through our own life experiences and I'm so thankful for my gospel knowledge.

I reached a point, finally, where I felt like *everything* having to do with cancer was behind me once and for all. I thought that day would never come. I'd had all my surgeries, except for a nipple reconstruction. I wasn't ready to face that one yet. I felt like I'd gone through enough for now. Chemo and radiation was behind me. I had hair again! My boys were into the "terrible twos." This posed equally demanding challenges as did the cancer. Let me just tell you about some of the things they did.

We'd bought great big bottles of pancake syrup. One day I fixed them pancakes and then ran downstairs for a few minutes. When I came back up they'd poured sticky syrup all over the dining room table. It had dripped down to the floor and on the chairs. They had literally rolled in it so they both were dripping with syrup from head to toe......

Another thing they loved to do was climb on the sink shelf in the kitchen, turn on the water and spray the kitchen and dining room with the sprayer. They got water *everywhere*! The walls, ceiling, floor, cupboards, drawers, countertops, -- it was awful!

They also tried to bathe the cat every chance they got. They'd catch him and force him into a tub of water. The poor cat didn't have a voice so it couldn't call for help. Luckily they never succeeded in drowning him.

One time they got into a 50 lb. bag of rice in my food storage, opened it up and threw rice everywhere. They also took my canning jars and used them for bowling pins.

We lived on a very busy street. The boys learned how to open the door and get outside. They would just take off! We didn't have our front yard fenced and I really worried about them getting hit by a car. So I had David put a lock way up high on the door that they couldn't reach. But the boys still kept getting out! I couldn't figure out how they were doing it so I spied on them. Those little monsters took a broom and used the handle to pop the lock up and then they could open the door!!

I begged David to fence the back yard. I thought if the back was fenced, then the boys could play out there safely. Wrong! They learned how to squeeze through a little tiny gap in the fence that led to the front yard, and they would escape through that!

One day I could not find either boy. I looked everywhere. I called the neighbors and nobody knew where they were. I ran outside and found Shane walking naked down the road -- it was really cold out too because it was fall. I scooped him up in a blanket and sat him in the house. I still couldn't find Scott. It had been almost an hour. I called my mom and she told me to call the police. I did. I then felt prompted to go next door to the neighbor's barn. There was a huge horse, like a Clydesdale, you know, those great big ones? And standing right beneath him was my Scotty! I was petrified. I mean that horse could kick him, or something and Scott would be toast. But it was really weird. It was like the horse knew that something was up and he stood perfectly still. I got Scott to come out -- after much coaxing -- and when I did the police had shown up. It ended happily.

It wasn't that my boys were brats or that I was a bad mother. They were very busy little twins and were curious. It took turning my back for just a second to have disaster strike. It was hard to discipline them because they had their own twin language and didn't communicate like other children. I hadn't even realized it until I saw a home movie of the girls at their age and saw they were talking up a storm. I had them tested and we learned that they were very smart, but just developmentally delayed in communication.

CHAPTER SEVENTEEN

"Life Goes On"

Feeling that I'd closed the cancer chapter in my life, I reflected on how precious each new day was. It's interesting how people get caught up in the stupid things and forget what is really important. Having cancer opened my eyes and brought into focus what really mattered. I saw the real treasures of life -- my family.

I felt an urgency to get busy and accomplish some important goals I had set for myself. Many of the things had been postponed for the past few years because of my illness. I loved to be of service to others so I got involved in various projects. I started a food storage group in my ward and arranged all the cannery assignments. I did it for me as much as for everybody else. I knew if other people were depending on me to do it I would be more likely to get it done. I also volunteered as Room Mother for both Angie and Jessica's classes at school. I planned the parties and went on field trips. I also became a Reach to Recovery volunteer. I would go out and talk to newly diagnosed patients. I made a lot of friends doing that -- but I also lost a lot of friends -- to cancer. I guess that is what happens when you hang around people with cancer. Some of them don't make it.

I continued to do hair at home. I also started selling custom blinds and window treatments. On top of all this a friend asked me if I'd be interested in cutting hair at the Utah Boys Ranch a few hours a week. I said sure. I really enjoyed it too. Those boys were very troubled and needed to feel somebody cared about them. I found I really did. I was sort of like a mom to them.

The American Cancer Society did a feature story on me with their annual report, complete with photographs. I also did an interview for a local radio station. I did a couple of fashion shows as a model for "Life After Breast Cancer." Joslyn and I started doing fireside talks at many different wards around the valley. We'd discuss our cancer experiences and hand out shower card packets explaining how to do monthly self exams. We felt it was important for women to know that cancer can happen to anyone -- it doesn't discriminate. Early detection can save your life.

Time passed, and every few months I had to go in for blood tests and chest x-rays. They usually turned out normal. Except one time the x-ray showed a spot on my lung.

"It may be nothing," the doctor said, "It's probably scar tissue but we'll want to take another picture in a few weeks to see if it's changed." I spent the next few weeks worrying that the cancer had come back.

The second x-ray showed the spot was still there and possibly bigger than before. I was so scared. *I don't want to go through this again!* I cried to the Lord. *Please don't let me reoccur.*

My family and ward held a special fast for me. The next x-ray was clear. The spot was completely gone. The doctor couldn't believe it. I even saw the spot myself on the other x-rays, but this one was normal. I made it through another trial!

In December of 1994 I decided to go ahead and have the surgery for nipple reconstruction. I also decided to lower the implant a little because it was kind of high and didn't look quite right. They took a skin graft from the inside of my thigh to construct the nipple and then they tattooed the areola. After that I felt almost normal again and I looked really good in a bathing suit.

CHAPTER EIGHTEEN

"Beginnings and Endings"

I'd been told that my chemotherapy would cause me to go into menopause but actually the opposite happened. My usually erratic cycle became regular as clockwork. In January of 1995 I found myself plagued by nausea and fatigue. I wondered if I might be pregnant again. Two urine tests came up negative but the symptoms persisted so I had a blood test.

It was positive! I was pregnant!

I told my oncologist and she was *not* happy with the news. She recommended an abortion but I was totally against it. I did worry about my cancer recurring, but I'd never give up my baby.

The timing of this pregnancy was not great. I'd just started tending my nephew Taylor full time and I still had both of my twins at home. I was excited though because in my mind I thought that if Heavenly Father wanted me to have another baby then I must be okay.

David had a hard time accepting it. I think he had a strong fear that my cancer would come back too. My doctor kept saying the pregnancy with the twins did not CAUSE the cancer, but it may have accelerated it because my cancer was what they call "estrogen positive." The pregnancy raised the estrogen levels in my body which caused the cancer to grow more rapidly. At least that was how it was explained to me. However, as far as medical science was concerned I was now considered cancer free.

We still needed to be concerned about the damage the chemotherapy might have done to my body and whether that would affect my ability to carry the baby.

I went in to see my OB -- Dr. Curtis. He was rather surprised with the news of my pregnancy too. He placed the obstetrical stethoscope on my stomach and listened for a long time. He couldn't hear anything. He checked my chart to see how far along I was.

"Well, you may not be along quite far enough to pick up the heartbeat. We'll just try it again at your next appointment."

This was in February, so I made an appointment for March 7. In the meantime I was soooooo sick. This pregnancy was worse than any of the others. I was sure it was because I was now in my thirties, and my body had been through so much. My stomach was getting bigger and sometimes I thought I felt little flutterings even though I knew it was probably too early for that. I was due in early September. I went shopping and bought maternity clothes and baby things. I planned out how to decorate the baby's room. My girls were really excited to have a baby coming.

I hated to admit it, but something didn't feel right. I had feelings of trepidation about going to see the doctor in March. I had nightmares that my baby was dead. Every time I planned what kinds of things I wanted to buy to decorate the baby's room it was like a little voice told me not to do it. But I didn't have a miscarriage so I assumed everything was okay.

As March 7 drew closer the feelings of fear increased. I was approximately 14 weeks along. I asked my sister-in-law Michelle (who was also pregnant and due two weeks ahead of me) to come with me to the doctors because if something *was* wrong I didn't want to get the news alone. She said okay. We sat in the examination room and I laid back on the table while Dr. Curtis tried again to find a heartbeat. He switched on the machine and I could hear a strong 'swish, swish, swish' and I thought, *Oh good, everything is okay.* But then he said, "Well, that is *your* heartbeat and the placenta sounds healthy. Let's see if we can find baby."

He moved the amplifier all over my stomach, listening... listening... the minutes passed and he made comments about how the baby could be turned, or the placenta could attach itself in such a way as to muffle the heartbeat. But inside, my heart sank. I knew something was wrong.

"Am I really pregnant?" I asked because I'd heard of people having "hysterical" pregnancies where they show all the symptoms but they really aren't.

"Oh, yes," he confirmed, "your pregnancy test was positive, no doubt about that."

He sent me downstairs for an ultrasound. I looked at my stomach thinking, *I look pregnant. Why do I have to go through this? Can't I just have a normal pregnancy after all I've been through?*

The technologist came in and scanned my stomach, moving all over the place but nothing was showing up on the screen. Michelle had been watching very closely and made the comment, "There isn't any baby there." The tech quickly said, "Oh, I'm sure there's a baby, but I think I need to do a vaginal scan to get a better look."

She performed an internal ultrasound (that was an experience I don't care to relate). Finally she stopped and looked at a little black spot on the screen and asked, "How far along are you?"

"About 14 weeks," I replied.

She was really quiet for a few seconds and then she said, "Well, I'm really sorry to tell you this, but it looks like your baby died at about 6 weeks gestation."

I just burst out bawling. *My baby was dead.* I couldn't believe it. *Why didn't I have a miscarriage?* I had been carrying a *dead baby* inside of me for *seven weeks* and the thought of that just freaked me out. I wanted it *out* --- now.

I had to go back upstairs to Dr. Curtis and discuss my "options."

"Well, we can do one of two things," he explained, "you can wait for your body to miscarry it naturally, or I can perform a D&C."

"Can you do the D&C tonight?" I asked.

He checked with his nurse and came back with "Sure, we can do that tonight."

"Then do it --- right away."

149

I found a telephone in the hallway and called my mom's house. Angie answered. I told her the baby was dead and she fell apart. She'd been so anxious for this baby to come. She'd picked names and everything. I wished I could have told her in person instead of on the phone but I was too upset to think straight. I called David because I wanted him to be with me. He came to the hospital and waited till it was time for the surgery.

As we drove home after the D&C we were both unusually quiet.

"I'm sorry," David said, "How do you feel now? Are we done having kids?"

"I don't know," I answered, "I have to pray about it."

He sighed.

I went through a lot of grieving over the loss of that baby. I didn't know what Heavenly Father was trying to tell me. Was this to tell me there were more kids for us but now wasn't the time? Or was the death a sign that I should NOT have any more children? I was so confused and I had no clue what to do. David wanted me to call a doctor and make an appointment for him to get a vasectomy. I was not comfortable with that decision. All I could think about was:

What if I die, and David remarries someone who wants to have a baby with him? I know he thinks he doesn't want more, but if that situation comes up, he might feel differently. I can't be responsible for doing anything that would prevent that.

This turmoil continued for weeks. I prayed so hard to know and understand Heavenly Father's will. I went to the temple and pondered over it. I wanted to do what was right. I had many things to consider: my health, David's wishes, and what I believed about the gospel and raising families. To me it wasn't a big deal to have more, but I knew it was to David and I respected his feelings.

In July I was doing a breast exam and all of a sudden I realized I felt a lump in my other breast -- the one that didn't have cancer before. It was a heart stopping moment. *Oh no, I've recurred*, I thought. I made an appointment with my oncologist immediately.

"It appears to be nothing to worry about," said Dr. Legant. "It's just fibrous tissue. Normal lumps that women get."

"Oh, hurray!" I breathed a sigh of relief.

Shortly after that I got called as a counselor in the Primary Presidency. I thought, *Oh good -- Heavenly Father wouldn't call me to this position if I was just going to die in a few months.*

In August I received an answer to my prayers about having another baby. I came to the realization that my family was complete and I wasn't supposed to have any more kids. I was a little bit sad, but mostly I accepted it just fine. I felt very peaceful about it. But for some reason, I *still* was *not* comfortable with David having a vasectomy.

CHAPTER NINETEEN

"Queen of Denial"

Nearly five years had passed since I was first diagnosed with cancer. Sometime in October of 1996, I started feeling bad again. I was extremely dizzy and sick to my stomach. My arms and legs would go numb a lot. I was tired all of the time. But I tried to ignore it. At first I thought I had the flu because the kids had been sick and throwing up. We had a family Halloween party and I felt so sick I didn't enjoy it at all. I went in for a blood test to see if I was pregnant again, but it was negative. The holidays were approaching and I wanted a little extra money for Christmas so I took a job at Southtown Mall working for Western Nut company. I was still cutting hair at the Boys Ranch too. I was working those outside jobs, tending my nephew Taylor, cutting hair, serving in Primary, doing the food storage group --- no wonder I was tired!!

In November, around Thanksgiving I still felt sick. I knew then that it had to be something more than the flu. People kept telling me I was doing too much and I was running myself down. I tried taking vitamins but it didn't help me feel any better. I thought I should go see the doctor, but that intuitive voice warned me it was going to be bad news and I was too afraid to hear it. I didn't want anything to spoil the holidays. I decided to wait until the new year --- you know, the old denial thing. I was almost at the five year mark of being cancer free and I didn't want to be paranoid about it.

In October I learned that Joslyn's cancer had come back. She had ten brain tumors and was given only a few months to live. I was devastated. She and I talked a lot, and cried a lot. I was so upset about her that I was afraid I was having "sympathy" sickness. I remember one day I went to the temple. As I was coming out of the locker room there stood Joslyn... all dressed in white like I was. It startled me. For a split second I felt like I had entered heaven and she was there to greet me. We were both so emotional we started crying. We sat beside each other through the session and wept through the whole thing.

Christmas came and went. I *still* felt awful. I was nauseous and dizzy *all* of the time. I'd fall asleep sometimes in the middle of the day because I just couldn't stay awake. I had another pregnancy test and it too, was negative. So I forced myself to see Dr. Legant in January. She took a blood test and told me everything looked good. But I was laying on the exam table in her office so sick I could hardly move and I said, "I *know* that something is *wrong* because I feel like I am going to die." She asked me if I wanted her to do a CT scan or MRI but I said no. I thought, "If my blood work looks good, then why waste the money on the scan?" So I went home.

On January 15, 1997 Annette was so sick that she could not get out of bed. She hadn't eaten in three days. If she stood up she became so dizzy she thought she might faint. She couldn't even walk. She kept the kids home from school that day so they could take care of her.

She and I were talking on the phone that morning. Annette sounded awful. We tried to figure out what could be wrong with her. Suddenly the conversation took a turn right into the twilight zone. Annette was not making sense and she kept laughing and rambling on and on. I realized something was not right.

"Annette, are you okay?" I asked.

"No," she replied.

"Is someone there with you?"

"Yes."

Annette would then act like she was trying to carry on a trivial conversation like you would if someone was there and you wanted the person on the phone to realize you were in trouble without "the bad guy" suspecting it. I began to get really nervous. I knew that since Annette was a beautician there were people in and out of her house all the time. Maybe some guy was there trying to hurt her.

"Annette, is somebody there trying to hurt you?" I demanded.

"Yes, um... the doctor, uh... was trying to figure

out... yeah, right, that's it. Uh huh."

"Annette! I'm not kidding -- is there somebody there trying to hurt you?"

"Yes, you're right, that's it."

I wasn't sure I was hearing correctly and my stomach was getting sick.

"Annette," I said very sternly, " Is there a man there who is trying to hurt you?"

"Uh huh, yup."

"Do you want me to call the police?" I asked in terror.

"Well... the doctor said, um... right... haha."

She wasn't making any sense at all. I had horrible images flashing through my mind that some lunatic was there beside her waiting to hurt her when she hung up the phone and that Annette was trying desperately to get a message of help through to me.

All of a sudden I heard the phone fall to the floor with a thud and Annette screamed. Then the sound of the kids screaming bloody murder. "MOMMY! MOMMY! MOMMY!" they shrieked, "Are you okay? Mommy are you okay?"

All I could hear were those terrified screams, crying and chaos. I couldn't breathe. I held the phone in horror wishing I could just jump through it. I prayed fervently for their safety as I ran to my other phone and dialed 911.

An ambulance was dispatched and rushed Annette to the hospital. Meanwhile I had called David and also Annette's mom to tell them what had happened. A few hours later Dave called from the hospital and the news was not good.... Apparently what I heard on the phone was Annette having a grand mal seizure. They had done a CT scan at the hospital and it showed Annette had eleven brain tumors. They gave her three months to live.....

"These brain tumors are inoperable," Dr. Legant explained, but we can do radiation on them to shrink them down as much as possible."

"Okay," I said. "I'll do radiation But is my hair gonna fall out again?" I knew Joslyn had lost her hair but she'd had a different type of radiation.

"Yes, I'm afraid so," Dr. Legant answered.

"It figures," I sighed, "and I just got it colored too!"

Then I remembered something and moaned.

"What's wrong Annette?"

"I'll have to buy another wig!" I wailed, "I cut up my other one and colored it green for David's Beetlejuice costume last Halloween!"

You should have heard the laughter......

When Joslyn heard about me she started looking into all kinds of alternative treatments that we could try. She wanted me to go to Texas with her because some doctor there was trying an experimental treatment for people with inoperable brain tumors. Joslyn had had a few months to think about things and she knew she was dying so she was fighting as hard as she could to live. She tried a juice fast to clean out her insides and detoxify her body. She drank nothing but juice for weeks. I don't think it helped. She was looking on the internet for the latest treatments. She wanted me to drink wheat grass (which I tried but it was awful) and take shark cartilage and all kinds of weird things.

David told me to stick to what the doctor said not get into all this strange stuff. His attitude was, "Let Joslyn try it first and if it works for her then you can do it if you want."

I understood how Joslyn felt. When you know you're dying you panic and you try to believe all the home remedies will help. I had lots of people telling me to take this vitamin and that herb. Drink this concoction and eat that. I know they meant well. I appreciated all their concern, but I knew it was too late for me. The Spirit told me in the hospital that my time was limited. I knew I was going to die. And the funny thing was that I accepted it. I was at peace. I didn't have to fight it anymore. I had done *everything* I possibly could with faith and modern medicine to live. The scriptures say that you can be healed by faith if you're not appointed unto death. So now I knew, it was my time to go and that was that. You can't change Heavenly Father's time table.

I went through two weeks of radiation and the horrible vertigo and nausea subsided only slightly. The radiation would keep working for several weeks after treatments stopped so they planned to do another MRI in March or April. I hoped I'd be around then.

It's weird to think about the future when you know you're dying. Jessica would be turning eight years old in March. Would I be here to see her baptized? I would be turning 34 in May -- or maybe not. Who would die first? Me, or Joslyn? My boys would be starting kindergarten this year. I really felt that I had to get them in school before I could die. That was my goal. That is what I focused all my energy on. I'd try to make it to that point. They would be starting school in July. But I was told I'd only live until April. I left that up to Heavenly Father.

David's dad came out to stay with us at the end of January. I was not supposed to be left alone in case I had another seizure. I was on Dilantin which is an anti-seizure pill but we didn't know if the dosage was sufficient yet. All of my driving privileges were revoked so I had to be chauffeured around. I was in no shape to take care of the kids and the house by myself. Dad had just retired in December, so in an odd twist of fate this was perfect timing for him. We appreciated him so much. He came in and really took over. He was wonderful to all of us. We became very dependent on him.

Every morning before I got up Dad made sure I drank a glass of *Shaklee Instant Protein*. It really helped give me the energy I needed to get of bed. It also helped with the nausea.

Because I knew my time was short, and things could go downhill rapidly I was determined to set and meet some important goals. First of all I wanted to complete photo albums for each of my children; one for David and one that would be a family album. With the help of friends I met that goal.

I also wanted to write letters to each of my children for important events in their lives such as birthdays, high school graduation, missions, and weddings. I found I couldn't write them myself because of weakness in my hands, so I recorded them and had my sister-in-law Michelle type them up. It was so hard to do those letters. I would start to cry and have to turn off the recorder. I wanted so much to be here for all those events! Telling my daughters how much I would miss not helping them out with their weddings -- telling the boys that I hoped they would remember me because they were so young when I died.... it was really hard for me to do it. But it was so important because I hope those letters will mean a lot to them and I wanted them to have something from me on those special days.

My mom and I picked out a pattern and material for her to make a dress for me to be buried in. It was a long white dress with lots of lace. I had Olan Mills take a picture of me in it for her because I wanted her to have a picture of the dress -- it was probably the most beautiful one she ever made. She had bought me all of my temple robes for a present the previous Christmas. She had no clue at the time she was buying them that they were for me to be buried in.

I started to lose my hair again so I put it into several braids and cut them off. Then I let Jessica shave my head. It wasn't such a big deal this time. Joslyn came over and we took the braids, put ribbon on them, and attached a card with a special saying for each of the kids and one for David. Joslyn and I still tried to maintain our sense of humor. I used to tell the people that the first thing I was going to do when I got to the "other side" was take a peek down my dress to see if I had a breast... and then I hoped there were mirrors in heaven cause I wanted to know my hair was there!

I got to say goodbye to a lot of people. When the word got out that I had so little time left everybody wanted to see me. My old friends from high school had a luncheon for me. People from my other wards held parties. The American Cancer Society presented with me a plaque for my work in the Reach to Recovery program. There were different fund raising events to help with medical and funeral expenses. Airline tickets were offered to us to go on a "last" family vacation wherever we wanted.

"How about Disneyland or Hawaii?" someone suggested.

"No, I want to go to Michigan to visit David's mom and dad." I said. (Dad had gone home for a few weeks)

So Michigan is where we went. I brought dried flowers to make a floral arrangement to go in their family room. When I was there I saw they had a great big window like mine so I offered to make them drapes. I wanted something for them to remember me by. Saying goodbye at the airport was really hard. I gave mom a big hug and said "Well, this is probably the last time I'll see you... in this life. Just know that I love you."

I don't think she had prepared for the reality of that goodbye because it hit her hard. A lot of people in my situation wouldn't say things like that. But I told it like it was. I didn't want to go with any regrets for not saying what was in my heart.

People gave me tapes of music to listen to and one that was my favorite is by Hilary Weeks and it's called "He Hears Me." There's one particular song on there that I listened to called "Be Still." When I heard this song I immediately thought of Joslyn.

"This is *our song*! I thought. I felt I had to hurry and play it for her. She was very ill and wasn't seeing visitors but I found David and said, "Hurry, you have to take me to Joslyn's right now!"

I guess I sounded pretty desperate because he didn't ask questions. He pulled up in front of her house.

"I won't be long. Just wait here for me," I told him.

I knew Joslyn didn't have much time left. We'd spoken on the phone a few times recently and she knew it was getting close. When she had first recurred I joked to her, "Don't be calling me as your mission companion when you get to the spirit world!" Now that we were both dying I felt that was exactly what was happening.

The closer Joslyn got to leaving this life the more afraid she became. She felt like her faith was wavering and she had started questioning everything she once thought she believed.

I knocked on the door and asked to see Joslyn. I told her I had to play a song on the tape for her. She said the tape player was in the family room. We went in there and she was so sick she was on her knees. I got down on my knees too, and together we listened to the words of the song:

Woman's Voice:
Another day, I'll try again
But can you tell me, will the hurting ever end?
I've been taught and I believe
But it's been awhile since I've been on my knees
And I need You by my side
I don't have the strength to make it on my own
And Lord, do You hear my prayer?
How soon will you answer me?

Man's Voice:
I know you're weary. I know you've had all you can bear

There's Always a Rainbow

And now you come to me, on bended knee
I promise I'll be there.
I've watched you struggle, and yet I can see how much you've grown
Child could you feel my power, in your darkest hour
You were not alone.
Be still and know that I am God
I'm by your side, whom shall you fear
I'll give you strength, my child I am here
Be still and know that I am God
And there's no prayer, that I can't hear
Lift up your head. My child
I am here.
© Hilary Weeks
"He Hears Me"

We listened to this song, held each other and bawled. I had a strong feeling that it was the last time I would ever see her alive. And it was. She passed away in her sleep, at home on May 13, 1997. Two days before my birthday.

I was really upset when Joslyn died. It's so hard to lose a friend anyway, but when you know that your turn is coming it is even scarier. I went to her funeral and it was beautiful. I could feel Joslyn's presence in that chapel. It was so strong. I wasn't feeling well so I didn't go to the cemetery but I asked her husband Joel if I could take some of the flowers from the graveside to dry and make an arrangement for him. He said okay so I went later on in the day. When I got to the cemetery I stood by her grave and I freaked out. I kept thinking, "Joslyn is here, *all alone* in this cemetery. I can't leave her here all by herself!" I was having an anxiety attack about leaving her. I had to go home and take an anti-anxiety pill because I was so sick over it. I am sure this had more to do with my fear of being alone than it did with her. I kept thinking I heard her voice in my head saying, "It's okay Annette, I'm not really *there*." But I was too stressed to pay attention to it.

CHAPTER TWENTY

"Packing Up, Moving On"

I had good days and I had bad days. I was *always* nauseated. That never went away. I tried not to complain too much. I had very little pain in my head, (with 11 brain tumors you'd think I'd have headaches but I really didn't.) Mostly my discomfort concentrated itself in my back, ovaries, liver and down my legs. A bone scan showed something on my spine and ribs but no one confirmed if it was cancer or not. I believed it was. An ultrasound of my ovaries showed they were abnormally large. I felt like the cancer was spreading *everywhere*. I'd heard that still small voice so often in the past that I could now easily recognize it. I'd learned to trust my feelings and instinct.

I had another MRI on March 27. Nine of the brain tumors had shrunk so small that they looked like calcifications and the other two had shrunk considerably. Radiation had bought me some time.

The pain had increased considerably by the time we got back from our trip to Michigan. I was taking morphine every day. But despite all this, it was decided that we were going to have a temporary house guest.

David's grandma, who was also dying of cancer, came to stay with us for a week. Grandma was a very demanding person and difficult to deal with. But I didn't want her to stay in a hotel all alone. She was very sick. She was dying of cancer and I could relate to what she was going through. There was no way I was going to allow her to stay in a hotel all by herself with no one to help her. But even I was not aware of just how ill she was at the time.

The first couple of days after she arrived, she mostly slept because the trip from Ohio had taken a lot out of her. She then began to go downhill rapidly. Within another day she could no longer go to the bathroom by herself. I had to help her with this. I'm a really tiny person and Grandma was a big, heavy person. I had to do a lot of lifting and pulling. It was hurting me because I didn't have the strength to cope with this! Having her in our house was very stressful and the peace we'd had previously had vanished. Everyone was cranky and irritable. I wasn't sure I could deal with it for even one more day. I wasn't getting any sleep because she would call out for me in the middle of the night and I was afraid that I wouldn't hear her and she would fall trying to get out of bed. She had nightmares and woke up screaming and terrified. I would have to go in and calm her down, but then she wouldn't want me to leave. This kind of care giving is hard on a well person, never mind someone who is also dying of cancer!

Once I realized how close to death she was I was very glad to have been able to help her and have her there. I saw her personality change from a proud, independent woman to one with humility and appreciation. I felt that when I finally crossed over to the spirit world I would be given the job of teaching her the gospel because in this life she had no religious beliefs. She came to know I cared about her. Even though the experience was stressful I'm glad she hadn't stayed in Ohio where she might have died all alone. She arrived at my house the end of June and spent ten days with us before going into the hospital where she passed away on July 3, 1997.

By the end of July my own health was deteriorating rapidly and I decided it was time to start saying my goodbyes. I asked to be allowed to get up in sacrament meeting in my ward to thank everyone for all they had done and say goodbye. I played the tape of the song that Joslyn and I called "our song." I talked a little bit about some of the spiritual experiences I'd had. I don't think they'd ever had a sacrament "farewell" quite like that one before! Everyone was so quiet; you could hear a pin drop. No babies were even crying. It was totally silent.

I spent a weekend in Las Vegas with David visiting my grandparents. My sister Melanie and her husband Doug came with us. I was so afraid I was going to die the first night we were there. I felt so sick. I was afraid to fall asleep because I was sure I wouldn't wake up in the morning. I kept praying, *Please Heavenly Father, let me have one last weekend with my husband. Please don't let me die tonight.* I finally told David how I was feeling and he promised to listen for my breathing the rest of the night so I could get some sleep. The next morning I felt a little better and was able to enjoy the rest of the trip.

When we returned to Utah I stopped going out as much and stayed home most of the time. The kids went back to school. My boys started kindergarten. I'd realized my most far-reaching goal. I'd lived to see them go to school. Heavenly Father understood how important this had been to me. He'd given me more time. The doctor had said three months... but I was going on seven.

One day the phone rang. It was my sister-in-law Michelle.

"Annette, Michael is getting baptized on August 9th. I know that you don't know how you will be feeling by then, but if you can, would you give a talk at his baptism?"

"Yeah, I think I can do that," I answered. I wasn't sure if I could or not, but it was another goal to shoot for. Maybe I could just keep my calendar too full to work in dying.

In the time leading up to the baptism, which was only two weeks, I noticed I was having a terrible time concentrating and I couldn't remember things. My hands and legs were numb almost constantly and sometimes I couldn't even pick up the telephone. It was like my hand didn't belong to me. I really wanted to participate in Michael's baptism --- I knew it would be the last family event I ever attended. Somehow I willed myself to stay on top of it.

I made it through the baptism. I'd prepared the wrong talk, but I winged it. The day following the baptism, I couldn't get out of bed. I no longer had the strength. I felt my body shutting down.

It was then I resigned myself to the fact that I would never see my children grow up, graduate, go on missions, and get married. I accepted that it was my time to go and comforted myself in knowing that Heavenly Father never falls short. He never leaves us alone. He wouldn't take me from my family without providing a way for me to still watch them from a distance. I was still my children's mother. I would attend those important events; I just wouldn't be able to be seen. I hoped that David would find another wife. I wouldn't want him to be alone, raising the kids all by himself. My sister Melanie was renting out her basement apartment to a divorced woman with three children. Her name was Sheri. I happened to catch a glimpse of Sheri one day and I told some of my friends that I thought she'd be a good wife for David because she was petite and blonde like me and David likes that. They couldn't believe I would be trying to set my husband up before I even died! I guess maybe that does take "being prepared" a little too far, huh?

I spent some time reflecting on my life wondering if I was ready to meet God. Was I at peace with the choices I had made? Had I fulfilled the mission I was sent here to perform? Did I teach my children well enough so my influence would continue after I was gone? What would happen to my own brothers and sisters? I had been the glue in the family and now they would have to do things themselves. Would they drift apart? I hoped not. I hoped that my absence would make them cling more to each other. Family is all we've got, now and forever. I didn't want any empty chairs in heaven.....

On August 19, 1997 Annette went into the hospital. Her abdomen was swollen with fluid. She was weak, dizzy and tired of fighting. Her veins were so bad it took nurses four hours to get an IV into her. She was wheeled down to radiology for another MRI to see how the tumors were. They also did an ultrasound on her stomach. She was pretty much out of it and wasn't bothered by the procedures.

The tech told Annette's mother that the MRI looked the same as the last one. No change. The tumors were not growing. But it seemed obvious the cancer had spread throughout her body which is why she had the fluid in her abdomen. The pressure of this fluid pressed against Annette's ribcage, causing her to have trouble breathing. She tried to take deep breaths and couldn't. This often caused her to panic because she felt as if she were suffocating. Elevating her bed so she was in a sitting position helped to ease that somewhat.

The fluid from the IV began to infiltrate the surrounding tissues in her hand which made her hand swell up like a balloon. A decision was made to put a permanent catheter into her heart that would stay there "the rest of her life." It was horrible what she had to go through. It took two hours for them to put that in. At the same time, they stuck a tube down her throat and into her stomach to pump her stomach out because she kept vomiting. She was too weak to talk, and having the tube made it impossible anyway. She was hooked up to oxygen also, which she hated, so she kept pulling the tube away.

The pain got progressively worse. Annette's blood pressure was low. Morphine would decrease it further so they didn't give her any. Finally they gave her a pain patch which she wore on her back and it helped tremendously. She was much more quiet and comfortable after that.

The doctor continued ordering more tests.... a spinal tap, a bone scan... the family kept thinking, "Why bother? Why put her through this? We all know what is happening here. Just leave her alone! There's nothing more to do."

Annette was released from the hospital on August 27. She spent the next few days quietly at home with only immediate family.

Sunday morning came and Annette had what is called "the death rattle." It's a sound a person makes when they breathe, caused by fluid in the lungs. It usually signals death is very close. Her father-in-law knew when he heard it that she would be gone that day. He gathered up the children and took them to church, leaving Annette in the care of her husband and mother.

At approximately 1:50 pm, with David and her mom kneeling by her bedside, holding her hands, Annette's pain and struggles finally ceased. She just opened her eyes, gave a little gasp, and was gone. It was very peaceful.

Annette's brothers, sisters and in-laws arrived to pay their respects. Everyone knelt by her bedside as the bishop of their ward offered a beautiful prayer. He invoked the Lord to bless the house with Annette's presence for a few days that she might watch over her family during this difficult time. He blessed David to find the strength to handle everything. He also asked special blessings on the children.

Soon after the mortuary took her body away, the family members drifted back to their own homes to grieve. Her sister Michelle stayed behind to work on the obituary with Dave.

Soon, a knock came upon the door and a voice called, "You've got to see this!" Outside, over the house.... was a double rainbow! Everyone who saw it was sure Annette somehow put it there. She couldn't do just one rainbow either -- that isn't like her. She would go the extra mile and do two! This symbol had so much meaning to everyone who knew Annette. But it was especially comforting to her sister Michelle who had asked for a special sign to know that Annette was okay.

On Wednesday Annette's mom, mother-in-law, sisters, sisters-in-law and Angie went to the funeral home to prepare her body. They dressed her in the beautiful dress made by her mother, jewelry that had been given to her on her birthday especially for this purpose... her makeup was applied; her wig was combed and put on. She looked beautiful and even seemed to be smiling. Angie had brought some of Annette's perfume and sprayed a ton of it on her. It was bitter sweet to watch her spray Annette's pulse points.... knowing Annette no longer *had* pulse points.

Everyone knew Annette had touched many lives but none of us were prepared for the magnitude of the crowd that showed up to pay their respects. Nearly 700 people attended the viewing which lasted over 5 hours instead of the scheduled two. The line went down the hall, out the door and into the parking lot!

The next day nearly as many attended the funeral. There was a brief viewing an hour prior to services. About ten minutes before 11:00 the bishop invited all of the family to gather for a private goodbye. Everyone was given the chance to approach the casket and tell her farewell. David and the kids were last. David leaned down and tenderly gave her a goodbye kiss. Her mom and mother-in-law placed the veil on her head. David pulled the veil down over her face and the casket was closed.

As the casket was wheeled into the chapel, everyone rose to their feet in reverent silence. It was placed down front. On top of the casket was a spray of flowers that David had ordered. It contained one white rose for every year of Annette's life; four small red roses representing the kids, and one large red rose in the center which represented Dave.

The bishop gave the eulogy. There were three musical numbers, "The Test" (the song by Janice Kapp Perry that was one of Annette's favorites), "I'll Build You a Rainbow" and then David played "Looking Back" on the piano. That was also one of Annette's favorite songs.

It came time to go to the cemetery. The twins helped wheel their mommy's casket to the hearse. One on each side.... pushing ever so carefully. If only they understood the significance of their act.

It was a long drive to the cemetery and the roads that we took formed an upside down "L". As we turned onto the road where the cemetery was located I happened to look back behind us.... all the way down the road, as far as the eye could see, was a steady stream of cars with their lights on. My breath caught in my throat. Tears welled up in my eyes, spilling over my cheeks. Such a tribute to Annette! I hoped that wherever she was, she could see it.

At the cemetery the casket was carried over to the plot reserved for her. The lady from the mortuary was there and she explained that the casket would not be lowered into the ground until everyone had left. It's easier on the family not to see that. David's dad offered the dedicatory prayer on the grave. Everyone stood around, reluctant to leave. Knowing that once we did so, once we turned our backs and walked away it would be final. The door would be closed; and life would go on... without Annette.

Or would it?

After all, it was only her body being laid to rest. Her spirit, her essence, all that makes her what she is -- lives on. Annette did not cease to be. We know she is busily engaged in good works in the spirit world. We believe that because families are forever that this separation is only temporary. We know she is no longer in pain, no longer suffering the restrictions cancer put upon her. And because of who she is, we know, without any doubt, that her love for her family remains alive and that she continues to watch over them and is aware of their comings and goings.

In her own words, "I have a testimony and I know where I'm going. I'm not afraid to die ---

There's Always a Rainbow
I'm afraid of what I might have to go through to get there. I just don't want to fail the test."

POSTLUDE:

It's now the year 2004 and time for this book to come forth. A promise I made to Annette was that I'd be sure her story was published. Her patriarchal blessing said that she had "much to tell the world" and she wanted her cancer story to be shared. We worked on it together before she died, which is why it is mostly told in her own words.

I tried working on this manuscript several times in the six years since her death. But it always opened a wound that hadn't completely healed and I would re-live these experiences as if they had happened only yesterday. As time went on I sometimes thought maybe the opportunity to publish this book had come and gone and I'd missed it.

Just recently I had an experience that let me know Annette still wanted me to keep my promise and it was time to finish this book. So here it is, and hopefully it will find its way into the hands for which she intended it.

Oh yes... there's more to the story that I mustn't forget to include. Remember Annette thought her sister Melanie's tenant might "make David a good wife?" Apparently she was right! David and Sheri were sealed in the Manti temple in October 1999 . This formed a family with seven children between the two of them. Just this past year, sweet little Lukus was born making number 8!

And who doubts Annette was inspired when she said:

What if I die; and David remarries someone who wants to have a baby with him? I know he thinks he doesn't want more, but if that situation comes up, he might feel differently. I can't be responsible for doing anything that would prevent that.

Annette faced her cancer ordeal with wisdom, courage, and a deepened spirituality gained from learning to rely on her Heavenly Father for strength when all else failed. Her message to the world is to remember that no matter what trials are given to us.....

. . . ."there's *always* a rainbow

-------------------THE END---------------

About the Author

Michelle Kramer was born and raised in New England in the small town of Putney, Vermont. She was baptized into the Church of Jesus Christ of Latter-day Saints and moved to Utah in 1981. Michelle has had a life-long dream of becoming a published author.

Though *There's Always a Rainbow* is her first book, there are many more to come.

She is currently a Certified Medical Assistant specializing in obstetrics and gynecology.

She resides in Taylorsville, Utah with her four children and a mutt named Sweetie.